Aromatherapy
Made Easy

D1142753

Aromatherapy Made Easy

Simple Step-by-step Guide to Using Essential Oils

Christine Wildwood

Thorsons
An Imprint of HarperCollinsPublishers

Thorsons
An Imprint of HarperCollins*Publishers*
77–85 Fulham Palace Road,
Hammersmith, London W6 8JB

First published as *The Power of Holistic Aromatherapy* by Javelin Books 1996
Published as *Holistic Aromatherapy* by Thorsons 1992
This edition published by Thorsons 1997
1 3 5 7 9 10 8 6 4 2

© Christine Wildwood 1986, 1992, 1997

Christine Wildwood asserts the moral right to
be identified as the author of this work

A catalogue record for this book
is available from the British Library

ISBN 0 7225 3452 3

Printed in Great Britain by
Caledonian International Book Manufacturing, Glasgow

Contents

Conversions

5 millilitres	= 60 drops	= 1 teaspoon
15 millilitres	= 3 teaspoons	= 1 tablespoon
30 millilitres	= 2 tablespoons	= 1 fluid ounce
60 millilitres	= ¼ cup	= 2 fluid ounces
0.24 litres	= 1 cup	= 16 tablespoons
0.47 litres	= 2 cups	= 1 pint

Introduction

Aromatherapy is an aesthetic healing art which uses the essential oils extracted from various parts of aromatic plants and trees to promote health of body and serenity of mind. Although its roots lie buried in the depths of Egyptian antiquity, its principles are none the less valid today. Modern aromatherapy draws on the knowledge of several ancient healing arts which can sometimes include reflexology, shiatsu and other massage techniques as well as the skills passed on by the twentieth-century pioneers.

Aromatherapy can form part of a holistic healing regime as well as being a preventative therapy in its own right. It gives pleasure through the sense of touch (massage), the sense of smell (aromatic oils), the sense of sight (pleasant surroundings), and sometimes through the sense of hearing (soft music). By so doing, it helps to create favourable conditions in body and mind for healing to take place quite naturally.

This book sets out to explain aromatherapy simply and is meant as a guide for those wishing to use the art as an aid to promote health and vitality for themselves and their families. For those wishing to go deeper, I have listed some very good massage books and the addresses of one or two training establishments in the Appendix. The art of massage could not possibly be explained in a book of this size, but the simple techniques described in Chapter 4 will suffice for those intending to use aromatherapy as a self-help regime.

I have chosen to tread the holistic path, which means looking at the prevention and the possible causes of illness rather than attempting solely to quell the symptoms. Chapter 1 is devoted to this concept and I strongly urge the reader to study this before turning to Chapter 6, which deals with specific ailments.

Where appropriate, I have suggested other compatible therapies such as yoga, Alexander Technique (the re-education of posture), Bach Flower Remedies (for treating negative states of mind), and herbal medicine to enhance the treatment with essential oils. The only therapy that may be incompatible with aromatherapy is homoeopathy. Many homoeopaths are of the opinion that essential oils, particularly camphor, eucalyptus and peppermint, nullify the effects of homoeopathic remedies. If you are taking homoeopathic medicine, especially for a chronic complaint, it may be as well to avoid all contact with essential oils until your homoeopath gives you the all-clear.

Since this book was first published in 1985, the art of aromatherapy has truly blossomed. It has at last emerged from the wings into the limelight of popular awareness. The reason for its popularity is not too difficult to understand. Apart from the wonderful healing properties of essential oils, aroma-therapy massage is one of the most effective and enjoyable treatments available for soothing the detrimental effects of stress – or *distress*. Stress, in its many guises, accounts for the vast majority of illness in this world of speed, 'high tech' and emotional unrest. So may the art continue to thrive and bloom and restore the simple beauty and tranquillity of nature to the lives of each and every one of us.

IMPORTANT NOTICE

Information and suggestions in this book are meant as a guide. The reader is advised and encouraged to seek the aid of a qualified natural health practitioner, or a doctor of orthodox medicine, if under medication or suffering from long-term health problems.

Christine Wildwood 1992

1

The Holistic Approach

> The cure of the part should not be attempted without treatment of the whole, and also no attempt should be made to cure the body without the soul, and therefore if the head and body are to be well you must begin by curing the mind: that is the first thing . . . For this is the great error of our day in the treatment of the human body, that physicians separate the soul from the body.
>
> Plato, *Chronicles* 156 e

Plato wrote these words over two thousand years ago, yet he could very well have been describing the situation we have today. Some of us are only just beginning to open our eyes and are re-discovering the wisdom in these age-old words. In our new-found knowledge, we have coined the word 'holistic' to summarize this concept.

The word 'holistic' has its roots in the Greek *holos* which means 'whole'. In holistic healing, the whole person – mind, body and spirit – is taken into account. In all schools of natural healing, which includes aromatherapy, the most important underlying principle is that the body will heal itself if given the chance. This is achieved by sound nutrition, adequate exercise, sunshine, fresh air and, above all, by deep relaxation therapy or perhaps meditation to buffer the adverse effects of life's inevitable stresses and to counteract the potentially harmful effects of negative emotions. Body and mind are interrelated; whatever affects one will also affect the other. So a positive mental attitude is vital, for whole health is transient without it.

MIND

Even in orthodox circles, the idea that our state of mind and personality has an influence over our physical health is beginning to gain credence. For instance, there is a so-called 'cancer personality'. Such people give more than they take; they tend to hide their emotions and repress their desires just to please others. The 'migraine personality' is driven by guilt. These people are perfectionists, ambitious, hard-working and extremely neat and tidy. The 'eczema personality' is hypersensitive and, like the cancer victim, tends to repress his emotions. The 'heart attack personality' on the other hand, is aggressive, impatient, competitive and ambitious.

The great psychologist Carl Jung has written about the 'symbolism of illness'. He says that the *form* which an illness takes can be a reflection of the mental state. He cites examples of nausea with no apparent cause, where the patient is unconsciously saying 'I'm sick of this situation'. Another patient with inexplicable leg pains is saying 'I can't stand any more.'

In a wider sense, we must consider the effects of world issues such as damage to the environment by pollution of air, soil and water; the rapidly diminishing rain forests; wars, famine, and the nuclear threat. All of these issues can be a source of great emotional turmoil to some people.

The pressures of being poor, disabled, black, unemployed, or whatever, can lead to feelings of frustration, anger, resentment and depression. Such feelings almost inevitably lead to a breakdown of physical health.

Almost all of us can recall a period in our lives when we have been under physical and/or emotional stress and have become ill as a result. Perhaps it was just a cold, or possibly something more serious. Many people also become more accident-prone at such times.

Conversely, our physical state can influence our moods, behaviour patterns, and, in extreme cases, our sanity. Certain forms of schizophrenia can be triggered by food allergies to substances such as wheat gluten, caffeine, alcohol and chemical food additives.

An American, Dr David Hawkins, pioneered the use of megadoses of vitamins and a reformed diet to help control schizophrenia. Thousands of his patients have been helped, yet the attitude of the traditional psychiatrists remains sceptical.

Hyperactive children are also sensitive to certain foods and food additives – particularly to tartrazine, a dye used in orange squash and confectionery (although this has now been largely withdrawn as a food additive). The Hyperactive Children's Support Group has done a great deal of research amongst its own members, and have found that children improve on a wholefood diet as free as possible from chemical additives and refined sugar.

BODY

Aromatherapy, like all healing techniques, is a tool which can only serve to scratch the surface by relieving a few nagging symptoms, unless we go much deeper. In the end, true healing can only come from within. Aromatherapy will stimulate our own innate healing mechanism into action as well as soothing our troubled minds.

Before discussing aromatherapy in detail, we must first understand that we are each responsible for our own health and must decide to make the necessary changes in our attitudes, diet and life-style. It may not be as easy as swallowing a pill, but the reward will be an inner feeling of contentment and an outer aura of positive energy and vitality that can only come once we have restored our whole health balance.

Food and Drink

Let food be your medicine, and medicine your food.

Hippocrates

Food is an emotive subject; so many arguments rage as to what constitutes the 'ideal diet'. Is meat really good for us? Should we be vegetarian or even vegan? Or is the macrobiotic principle the ideal? My answer to these questions is that there is no one ideal diet suitable for all of us. We are each very different with varying needs. Whatever you believe about food, the only clear-cut rule, as far as I see it, is that our food should be as free as possible from harmful additives and the toxic chemical residues of modern farming methods – no easy task nowadays.

It may be relatively easy to buy organically-grown flour, but unsprayed, organically-grown fruit and vegetables are a rarity – unless you grow them yourself. Even when they are available from health food shops, they can be expensive; prohibitively so for some people. The best we can do at the moment, until the 'organic revolution' hits the high street, is to eat foods that are as near as possible to their natural state – not out of cans and packets whose contents have been doused in chemical additives. At least 50 per cent of our food should consist of raw or lightly-cooked vegetables and fruit. However, the very young and the very old cannot digest raw foods; so more home-made vegetable soups and fruit juices will provide the essential nutrients.

We should try to buy free-range eggs instead of battery eggs. Not only are they tastier but they will also be free of the residues of antibiotics and other chemicals added to the hen's diet to keep the poor creature 'healthy'.

According to Dr Michael Crawford of the Nuffield Laboratory of Comprehensive Medicine, battery eggs have twice as much saturated fat as free-range. A diet high in saturated fat (usually from animal source foods) is a contributing factor in heart disease. Health apart, the ethical reason for avoiding battery eggs should not be dismissed. This also applies to intensively-reared poultry and animals intended for food. Not only are they deprived of exercise, sunshine and fresh air, but they are also often pumped with 'therapeutic' drugs as well as growth-enhancing hormones. The toxic residues of these chemicals can end up in your body. So, free-range meat and poultry is preferable if you can find it.

Dairy products are not immune to chemical contamination. The most recent problem to come to light is iodine poisoning in people as a result of drinking milk containing unusually high concentrations of the mineral. Iodine is used to clean the cows' teats as well as the milking machines. It is also added to the winter fodder of dairy herds reared on iodine-deficient soils. Iodine-deficient cows tend to miscarry their calves. A far safer and ecologically sound alternative would be to dress the soil with composted seaweed; but, no doubt, the argument of 'cost effectiveness' would be sure to raise its head.

Convenience Foods

The modern food industry pours some three thousand chemicals into foods already tainted by chemical farming methods. Most of these substances are purely cosmetic – to 'improve' the colour, texture and flavour of canned and packaged foods. But none of these substances has been tested in relationship with the others as to the combined effect on body and mind. Nor is much thought given to the accumulative effect of these substances when ingested over a period of time, or even if the additives deemed safe today will be so tomorrow. The ban on the use of cyclamates (a type of sugar substitute) is a case in point. Furthermore, food additives are tested on animals, not people. The physiology of an animal is quite different from ours. Take carragheen moss for example; a harmless vegetable jellying agent to us, but it has been shown to cause ulcerative colitis in guinea pigs.

Food additives pose a lesser-known problem, namely that they add enormously to the burden placed on the liver and kidneys in eliminating them. We should all try to avoid food additives as far as possible, but people suffering from allergies, arthritis, kidney stones and urinary infections should avoid them like the plague.

Sugar

Most people now realise that sugar rots our teeth and can make us fat, but it has other hidden dangers as well.

1. The digestion of refined sugar is only possible with the aid of alkalising minerals and many of the B vitamins. Sugar does not possess such nutrients, so they must be drawn from the body's reserves, thus leaving a deficit.
2. Sugar increases the amount of uric acid in the blood which can lead to gout.
3. Excess sugar consumption is associated with artery disease leading to heart attacks.
4. It can cause hyperglycaemia (high blood sugar), hypoglycaemia (low blood sugar) and may eventually progress to diabetes.
5. Sugar can be addictive. When we eat sugar, the glucose level in the blood rapidly soars. The pancreas reacts by pouring high levels of insulin into the bloodstream to try to restore the blood sugar levels to normal. When we first eat sugar we experience a quick lift, but as soon as the blood sugar level stabilises, we feel hungry and depressed and reach for more sugar.

Many wholefooders believe that brown or raw sugar is better than white; but unfortunately it is almost as bad. It does contain a trace of the minerals and vitamins found in the sugar beet and sugar cane from which it is extracted, but it is still a highly-refined substance and can create the same metabolic disturbances as white sugar. The only slight advantage of raw sugar over white is that it is very bulky and strongly flavoured and possibly we automatically eat less of it.

Honey, *if used in small quantities*, is a much healthier

alternative to sugar. Honey contains two simple sugars, glucose
and fructose, which are easily digested. Fructose does not need
insulin for absorption, so a little honey can be taken by
diabetics. Honey has been eaten for thousands of years both
for pleasure and for healing. Incidentally, honey may not be
quite as detrimental to the teeth as sugar if used *sparingly*:
archaeological evidence suggests that tooth decay, despite
honey consumption, was quite rare in ancient times.

ALCOHOL
Alcohol in moderation, for example one glass of wine a day,
may actually be beneficial to health. It aids digestion by
encouraging the secretion of digestive juices. However, excess
alcohol can cause the same metabolic disturbances as sugar
and will eventually damage the liver. It is best to avoid it
altogether during pregnancy.

TEA, COFFEE AND COCOA
A healthy diet should really be totally free of these drinks.
Each contains caffeine - an addictive stimulant which acts on
the central nervous system - and oxalic acid which can
damage the kidneys and rob the body of calcium. Coffee can
be more damaging to the kidneys than the others because it
is diuretic (stimulates flow of urine) and is particularly harmful
to those suffering from irritations of the bladder and
enlargement of the prostate gland. Water decaffeinated (not
chemically treated) coffee is fine in small quantities, but still
contains oxalic acid, which is not good for the kidneys.
    The link between caffeine intake and anxiety symptoms is
well documented. If you find it difficult to give up caffeinated
drinks altogether, at least limit yourself to not more than three
small cups a day.

TWELVE STEPS TOWARDS A HEALTHIER DIET
The following is a general outline of a wholefood diet as
recommended by many nutritionists. It does not take into

account food allergies – some people are allergic to dairy foods or wheat for example – or whether you wish to avoid animal foods altogether. But it should serve as a useful guide that can be adapted to suit individual needs. Aim to alter your diet *gradually* over a period of six months. Drastic overnight changes will almost certainly lead to digestive upsets.

1. Buy organically-grown food if you can, but do not fret about it if you cannot.
2. Eat more wholemeal bread and other high-fibre foods such as dried beans, lentils, nuts, oats, brown rice and other wholegrain cereals.
3. Eat plenty of fresh fruit and vegetables – preferably unskinned, well scrubbed and raw in salads or lightly cooked.
4. Cut down on all fats, particularly those from animal sources such as lard, suet, butter, cream, full-fat cheeses. Use moderate amounts of cold-pressed oils such as virgin olive, sesame and sunflower seed (up to a tablespoonful daily).
5. Sweeten your food sparingly with honey or molasses, or more lavishly with dried fruits such as dates, figs and raisins.
6. Cut down on salt, even sea salt, and use more herbs to flavour your food.
7. Buy free-range eggs and poultry if possible.
8. Eat red meat only once a week if at all. Eat more fish, particularly oily fish such as mackerel.
9. Use skimmed milk and low-fat cheeses in place of the full-fat versions or substitute dairy milk with soya milk.
10. Avoid all processed foods in cans and packets that are laden with chemical additives.
11. Drink plenty of water (preferably bottled), herb teas and diluted fruit juices in place of ordinary tea and coffee.
12. Eat slowly in convivial surroundings, and, above all, enjoy your food.

Movement

The human body was designed to move. Unlike a machine that breaks down with use, we become stronger, more flexible and age more slowly if every muscle and joint is used frequently.

When we lived a simpler life we walked, swam, stretched and climbed as a matter of course almost every day of our lives. We did not consciously 'exercise' nor did we require supplementary exercise to keep our bodies finely tuned.

In relation to stress of any nature, whether it be the result of 'overload' or perhaps born of monotony, regular exercise increases the circulation, which in turn increases oxygen levels in the blood. This has a positive effect on our state of mind, bringing enhanced mental energy and concentration, the ability to sleep more deeply and a feeling of well-being.

However, natural movement which is also a pleasure rather than a chore is infinitely superior to indoor exercises with weights, or exercise that is so taxing that one aches from head to toe afterwards as a result of 'the burn'. Jogging is not a particularly good form of exercise either, especially on city pavements; all that pounding can put a great strain on the lower back and can damage the knees. Swimming, walking and dancing are arguably the most natural and enjoyable forms of movement, or you may prefer yoga, which is a good all-rounder, embracing body, mind and spirit. Try to find out about classes in your area.

However, if you are elderly, physically disabled or too ill to take much exercise, regular aromatherapy massage can be of enormous benefit, and it need not be carried out by a professional. Sensitive, nurturing massage given by a friend or a loved one can work wonders. While it cannot totally replace physical activity, it is in fact similar in body stimulation terms as twenty minutes of jogging! Moreover, the benefits to mind and spirit are immeasurable: tender loving care is the most potent healing force of all.

Light

Light is as much a nutrient as food and water, yet few of us even realize it. It is absorbed by our bodies and used in a wide range of metabolic processes. But artificial light is vastly inferior, lacking the full spectrum of the ultra-violet rays of daylight, and has been blamed for a number of ailments suffered by indoor workers. The most common problems associated with full spectrum light deprivation are lethargy, headaches, irritability, lack of concentration and a seasonal mental state known as 'winter depression'.

Light manufacturers have taken notice of reports about the importance of full-spectrum lighting and have introduced lights that simulate natural sunshine. They cost much more than fluorescent strips but last longer.

Light has two types of effects on us: a direct effect that causes a photo-chemical response in the skin – tanning and the formation of vitamin D from ergosterol; and an indirect effect through photoreceptors in our eyes. The type and quality of light entering our eyes can affect our hormonal balance and body chemistry as a whole, influencing our energy levels and the way we feel. The photoreceptors are part of a nerve network which lead directly to the hypothalamus – a portion of the brain controlling numerous physical and emotional responses directly and indirectly via the 'master gland' or the pituitary itself which governs the entire endocrine system. The same nerve network triggers the pineal body, the brain's little-used 'third eye', which is believed to be involved in the formation of chemicals used to transmit messages between brain and body. In Eastern philosophy, the third eye is a very important chakra (energy) centre for our spiritual development.

If it is a lovely warm summer's day as you read this, think before you go rushing out in the midday sun; bear in mind that a little of the sun's powerful energy is good, but too much can damage the skin resulting in premature ageing. So treat the sun with the respect afforded by the ancients. First protect your skin from the drying effects of the sun by applying a good moisturizing sun preparation or one of the sun protective oils described under 'Recipes' in Chapter 5. Start with as little as ten minutes' exposure the first day and build up the time gradually until you can spend half an hour in the sun, or an hour at the very most, without burning. There is no need to fry your skin to a mahogany hue; in fact, a very deep tan can rob the body of vital nutrients, particularly vitamin C and B-complex. People with very fair or sensitive skins may not be able to sunbathe at all. However, they will benefit from the energizing effects of the sun even if covered from head to toe in thin cotton garments that allow enough of the ultra-violet rays through without burning the skin.

The morning rays are said by yogis to be highly charged with prana (life force) and are the most beneficial to health. Even on a scientific level, the longer waves of ultra-violet light before noon and after four in the afternoon, are less likely to burn. So, in very hot summers, take your sun bath very early or very late in the day.

In the winter it is even more important to get outside for at least an hour a day. Surprisingly, the skin of the face and hands of white people has become super-efficient at absorbing ultra-violet rays. As little as twenty minutes' exposure can supply the minimum level of vitamin D required for a whole day's quota. However, dark-skinned people require much more light than this to maintain adequate levels of vitamin D.

Fresh Air

Air, like light, is a nutrient, but so vital that it is only possible to live for a few minutes without it. We all know how essential oxygen is for the lungs and the whole organism, but few of us remember that the skin also needs air as a stimulus for its normal functioning. It has sometimes been referred to as 'the third lung'. You may have heard the horrific tale of the small boy who was painted from head to toe with a metallic based substance for a carnival and who consequently died of respiratory failure.

Most people cover their bodies with layers of synthetic fibres that trap air and hinder the skin's natural metabolism. Clothes should ideally be of cotton and other natural fibres such as linen and wool as they allow perspiration to evaporate by the free-flow of air they afford.

Clean air is hard to come by today, especially if you live in a city. Whenever possible, visit the seaside and breathe in the bracing sea air. It is charged with negative ions which generate a feeling of well-being. The clean crisp air of mountainous regions is perhaps the most beneficial of all. But do not despair if you live miles from the sea and mountains; take a daily walk in your local park and as many trips to the countryside as you possibly can and breathe deeply.

These precious moments of breathing in the scents of grass, trees and flowers will help to bring about a state of harmony to a bustling mind.

Deep Breathing

Many of us are shallow breathers; we use only the upper part of our lungs, which means that toxic residues are not completely removed. As a result, the blood is deprived of much of the oxygen it needs to feed the body tissues, so we may end up feeling listless or suffer vagueness of thought. At the same time, the oxygen deficit hinders the assimilation of nutrients from the food we eat.

Ancient Oriental philosophies, such as yoga, recognise the importance of deep breathing for the maintenance of health. It is believed, in yoga, that special breathing techniques can extract from the air an etheric force known as prana (chi in Chinese philosophy). Prana is taken in with the breath and can also be absorbed in other ways, particularly through the skin. It recharges the whole organism: filling the body with vitality, facilitating clarity of thought and at the same time calming the mind.

THE COMPLETE BREATH

The yoga 'complete breath' is one of the easiest ways to begin learning to use your lungs efficiently and is very helpful to those suffering from respiratory ailments such as hay fever, asthma, bronchitis and so forth.

1. Find a quiet, well-ventilated room and lie on the floor or a firm bed with your arms at your sides, a few inches away from your body, palms face down.
2. Close your eyes, begin to inhale through your nose very slowly. Expand your abdomen slightly, then pull the air up into the rib cage, and then your chest. Your abdomen will be automatically drawn in as the ribs move out and the chest expands. Hold for a few seconds.
3. Now begin to breathe out slowly through your nose in a smooth continuous flow until the abdomen is drawn in and the rib-cage and chest are relaxed. Hold for a few seconds before repeating two or three times.
4. Now breathe in slowly as you did in Step 1 but gradually raise your arms overhead in time with the inhalation until the backs of your hands touch the floor.
5. Hold your breath for ten seconds while you have a really good stretch.
6. Slowly breathe out as you bring your arms back down to your sides. Repeat two or three times.

SPIRIT

The spiritual aspect of our being is hard to define, but is tied up with our relationship with ourselves, with other people and with our sense of purpose and meaning. Without purpose we become depressed or apathetic; life then appears bleak or meaningless. Even when we do not follow a spiritual path in terms of a religious faith, we may in fact be realizing our purpose in some other way. It could be through music, or some other art form, no matter how humble, or simply through our work, family, relationships, or through a love of nature or of animals – or more actively perhaps by working towards the realization of an humanitarian or green ideal.

It is also true to say that the mind-body can either trap or liberate the spiritual aspect of 'self'. The condition we call spiritual imprisonment or freedom depends upon how we think and feel. We cannot always change our outer situation, but we can change our attitude to it, which makes all the difference in the world.

The two exercises which follow will help you to get in touch with your inner powers. By creating a peaceful space within your life, especially if your mind is usually in a turmoil, you will begin to tap a source of healing, a positive energy that will not only strengthen your immune system, but will enable you to become stronger and more resourceful in the face of adversity.

Deep Relaxation

The following technique is based on a therapy known as 'autogenics' which is used in self-hypnosis. As in the breathing exercise described earlier, it may be easier to record the directions on tape or get someone with a soothing voice to read them out to you. Try to practise twice a day, preferably on an empty stomach.

Find a quiet, well-ventilated room with pleasant surroundings where you will not be disturbed. To enhance the atmosphere, vapourize your favourite essential oil (instructions are on page 94).

1. Lie down on the floor supported by pillows if desired – one under your head and another under your knees, or lie on a firm bed.

2. Close your eyes, take one or two deep breaths and let out the air with a deep sigh.
3. Now become aware of your feet. Mentally tell them to let go and say to yourself silently: 'My feet are feeling heavy, heavy and warm, heavy and relaxed; they are sinking through the floor.' Allow enough time to experience the heaviness.
4. Now think of your ankles. 'My ankles are getting heavy, heavy and warm, warm and relaxed . . .'
5. Now think of your calves. 'My calves are getting heavier, heavier and warm, heavy and relaxed, they are sinking into the floor.'
6. Now your thighs. 'My thighs are getting heavy, heavy and warm, relaxed and heavy . . .'
7. Continue moving over your whole body instructing each part to become heavy, warm and relaxed. Do not forget your spine, hips, buttocks, abdomen and even your face, tongue, jaws and eyes.
8. When every part of you is warm and relaxed say: 'My whole body is still . . . and at peace . . . relaxed . . . relaxed . . . at peace . . . warm, peaceful . . . and relaxed.'

   At first you may feel rather silly talking to your body in this way, but, in time, it will become much easier to fall into deep relaxation in a matter of minutes; initially, however, allow yourself a good twenty minutes or more until you have mastered the technique. If a part of your body needs attention – maybe you have a headache or suffer from rheumatic aches and pains – think warmth into the area. In time, you will be able to feel actual heat or a tingling sensation.
9. When you feel it is time to come back, say to yourself: 'I am going to get up now and I will feel happy, refreshed and eager to face the day.' Open your eyes; take your time before getting up. Have a good stretch from fingertips to toes; roll over on your side; when you are ready, get up.

Meditation

One of the simplest ways to begin meditating is to be aware of your breath as you breathe in and out. Try to practise this exercise once or twice a day, preferably on an empty stomach.

1. Find a quiet place where you will not be disturbed - a pleasant room or outside in a garden or by a stream.
2. Sit on the floor or the ground if you can, but you may use a chair if you are more comfortable this way. There is no need to sit in the lotus position, but in a simple cross-leg pose. Sit upright without slouching to facilitate your breathing.
3. Close your eyes and take some deep breaths. Become aware of your abdomen as it rises and falls with each breath.
4. Breathe in through your nose, but do not force it; allow yourself to breathe slowly but naturally. With each out breath count silently to yourself. Breathe in and out and count 'one'; in and out again and count 'two' and so on up to ten. Count only on the out breath. Once you reach ten, go back to one again.

   If you lose count or thoughts come crowding your mind, gently push them aside and start again with one. As with all the other relaxation and breathing techniques, the more often you practise the easier they become.
5. After about ten minutes or so, stop. Very slowly bring back your consciousness into the present surroundings. Open your eyes, slowly stretch out your body and get up when you are ready.

Sleep

Sleep is nature's great restorer. It enables us to think and work to our utmost efficiency. The amount of sleep required by an individual varies. Some of us get by on four or five hours a night, others need eight or ten. Short sleepers tend to be easy-going extroverts, whereas those needing much more than eight hours a night are more likely to be introverted and creative. However, any adult who sleeps for ten hours or more *every* night is probably suffering from some form of reaction to stress and should look closely at their life-style, diet and emotions. Generally we need less sleep as we grow older.

THE PARTS THAT MAKE UP THE WHOLE

If you are experiencing difficulty in any of the key areas of life listed below, the chances are that you are not experiencing whole health. Many of these aspects are inter-related, and, as such, are not listed in any order of importance, nor is this list in any way comprehensive.

1. Eating and drinking: under-eating, over-eating, poor diet in general for whatever reason – choice, ignorance, poverty.
2. Breathing: polluted air, poor posture, smoking.
3. Elimination: constipation, catarrh, fluid retention, congested skin.
4. Personal hygiene.
5. Ecological and political: frustration, anger, despair.
6. Mobility: problems experienced by elderly or disabled people.
7. Controlling body temperature: problems of the elderly and the very young.
8. Communicating: speech impediment; problems experienced by people with learning difficulties.
9. Work: unemployment, stressful work, boredom.
10. Relationships: marriage, family, friends, workmates, loneliness.
11. Sexuality: especially problems of acceptance experienced by gay men and lesbians.
12. Money: poverty, debt, greed.
13. Other inequalities (real or imagined): being black, female, divorced, disabled, dissatisfied with appearance.

14. Play: no recreation/fun in life.
15. Freedom: imprisonment (jail), living under an oppressive regime.
16. Creativity/spirituality: no outlet for artistic expression/religious beliefs/humanitarian ideals.
17. Being divorced from nature: inability or unwillingness to see/touch/smell/experience the elements, flowers, trees, or to walk on earth, grass, sand.
18. Sleeping: broken sleep, insomnia, needing to sleep more than 10 hours *every* night, problems associated with shift work.
19. Environment: not only pollution, but dislike of one's surroundings at home or at work.
20. Death: fear of dying, inability to face up to the idea of death or bereavement.

CONCLUSION

It would be unrealistic, insulting, even ludicrous to suggest that a good organic diet and daily meditation is the answer to life's problems and that it will cocoon us in an etheric pink haze for the rest of our lives! What it *can* do is to buffer the adverse effects of life's inevitable stresses, enabling us to look at our problems objectively in order to seek an answer. It will help us to shake off minor ills and possibly prevent the development of chronic illness such as heart disease, high blood pressure, diabetes and the many other 'diseases of civilisation'.

In a much broader sense, people with a calm, positive and compassionate attitude to life are perhaps better equipped to help solve the many ecological, social and political problems facing the world today.

2

About Essential Oils

Essential oils, or essences as they are often called, are the basic raw materials of aromatherapy and perfumery. They have been poetically described as 'ethereal' or as the 'soul' of the plant. Other more down-to-earth people have described them in scientific similes: 'the plant's blood supply' or 'its hormones'.

In fact, essential oils are the odoriferous, volatile (they readily evaporate) liquid components of aromatic plants. They accumulate in specialized cells or in intercellular spaces in specific parts of the plant. They may be found in the petals (rose), the leaves (eucalyptus), the wood (sandalwood), the fruit (bergamot), seeds (caraway), roots (sassafras), rhizomes (ginger), resin (pine), roots of grasses (vetiver), and sometimes in more than one part of the plant. Lavender, for example, yields an essential oil from the flowers and leaves. The orange tree is particularly interesting for it produces three different- smelling essential oils with differing therapeutic properties: neroli (flowers), petit grain (leaves), and orange (skin of the fruit).

A plant produces essential oils for its own survival: to influence growth and reproduction; to attract pollinating insects; to repel predators; and to protect itself from disease.

The chemistry of essential oils is complex. They contain the plant's therapeutic properties in a concentrated form and are thus used in tiny amounts. Some of the main active constituents of essences include acids, esters, alcohols, aldehydes, phenols, acetones and terpenes. Some plants are named after their main chemical constituents. Vanilla, for example, is high in vanillin, geranium contains geraniol, camphene is found in camphor, and so forth.

Essences are technically classified as oils, but they are very different from ordinary vegetable or 'fixed oils' such as almond, soya and wheatgerm. Some have the consistency of water or alcohol; others are viscid. Because they are highly volatile, they do not leave a permanent mark on paper.

HOW ESSENTIAL OILS ARE EXTRACTED

The concentration of essential oils in plants is highest during warm weather and this is the best collecting time. However they are often so locked up within the plant cells that distillation of the plant is necessary to capture them.

The most classic method is direct distillation, which is a sophisticated process based on the Ancient Egyptian clay-pot method. Plant material is placed in the still and is in direct contact with the water. This is heated and the steam carries the essential oils into a condenser and then a separater. A far more efficient method, which prevents possible 'burning' of the distillate, is steam distillation. This is similar to the former method except that the plant material does not come into contact with the water; only the steam is passed over it.

The most recent innovation is vacuum distillation which is achieved at much lower temperatures, thus preserving the delicate flower fragrances more successfully. This method prevents the possibility of oxidation (exposure to the air) which can lead to rancidity.

Two outmoded methods of distillation (mentioned in many text books of aromatherapy and perfumery) were maceration (using heat) and enfleurage (cold). Vegetable oils or animal fats were used to absorb the essential oils which were then separated from the fat by alcohol. Essences readily dissolve in alcohol, but fat does not. The alcohol was later evaporated off, leaving the essential oil behind. This method was generally used to capture the essences of flowers such as jasmine and neroli whose fragrances would have been ruined by the intense heat of distillation. However, the high cost of this labour-intensive and time-consuming method has led to the wide use of solvents, such as petroleum ether, to extract the delicate flower essences. The solvents are separated from the essential oil by evaporation.

A relatively new, but at present, costly process of capturing precious fragrances is carbon dioxide extraction. This is of great interest to those who would prefer to avoid solvent-extracted 'absolutes'. Quite apart from concern over traces of solvent often left behind in absolutes, we cannot ignore the environmental effects of these substances being discharged into the atmosphere and possibly being absorbed by distillery workers. Carbon dioxide extraction is generally regarded as a cleaner alternative to the use of potentially toxic solvents.

The essential oil in citrus fruit is found in the outer rind, so simple pressure is the method used for extracting the oils. Although it was once carried out by hand, machines using centrifugal force are now used instead.

THE PROPERTIES OF ESSENTIAL OILS

All aromatic essences are endowed with antiseptic and bactericidal properties. Some have antibiotic and anti-viral properties as well – garlic and tea tree are the most powerful. Although the ancients may not have scientifically understood the reason why essences have the ability to heal wounds, to preserve flesh (mummification) and to help prevent the spread of infection (fumigation), empirical knowledge, the knowledge of experience, was proof enough.

Unlike chemical antiseptics, essential oils are harmless to tissue, yet they are powerful aggressors towards microbial germs. Dr Jean Valnet used essential oils to treat the horrific war wounds of soldiers during the Second World War. Not only did the fragrances of the essences cover up the putrid smells of gangrenous or cancerous wounds, but they also suppressed them altogether by retarding putrefaction.

Essential oils promote healing by stimulating and reinforcing the body's own mechanisms. Essences of camomile and thyme, for example, are credited with the ability to stimulate the production of white blood cells which help in our fight against disease.

Unlike pharmaceutical drugs, essential oils work with the body rather than against it. Drugs tend to suppress conditions without removing the cause. At the same time they induce poisons into the body which it then has to deal with as well as the illness.

Essential oils work more slowly than powerful drugs, but if used in the correct concentration side-effects are virtually non-existent. This also applies to herbal medicines which are often used in conjunction with aromatherapy.

To be fair to the orthodox profession, there must be a case for the occasional use of drugs; if, for example, a person fails to respond to natural treatment, or in 'life or death' situations, road accidents, or congenital organ malfunction where drug intervention may be vital.

THE SENSE OF SMELL AND ESSENTIAL OILS

Just how odours are perceived is a complicated procedure. The following explanation is the generally accepted theory at the moment. Odoriferous substances, such as essential oils, throw off molecules which are detected by the olfactory cells in the upper part of the nose. These cells are specialized sensory neurones embedded in a mucous membrane, each of which connects directly with the brain by means of a single long nerve fibre. Each cell body has a rod-like extension to the surface of the membrane, terminating in a brush of hair-like structures which are super-sensitive. Before an aromatic molecule can be detected, it must first be dissolved in the mucus. Responses to the aromatic molecule are then sent in the form of impulses via the nerve fibres to the olfactory area in the brain. Because the sensory processes/'hairs' are in *direct* contact with the source of smell, and because the olfactory cells connect *directly* with the brain, the sense of smell has a powerful and immediate effect.

This is because the area of the brain associated with smell is very closely connected with the limbic area of the brain which is concerned with our most subtle responses such as emotion, memory, sex-drive and intuition. The olfactory area of the brain also connects with the hypothalamus, a very important structure which controls the entire hormonal system by influencing the 'master gland' itself – the pituitary.

From this, we may conclude that any process which can send impulses directly to the brain can be used to influence the physical body and the emotions. For example, the aroma of hot food, especially when flavoured with herbs or spices, will stimulate the appetite by making one's mouth water and causing the digestive juices to flow.

Smell can sometimes evoke memories. Some people only have to take the faintest whiff of the entrance hall of a hospital to be sharply transported back in time to re-live a traumatic hospital experience; they may feel shaky or even nauseous.

Other aromas conjure up pleasant memories of first love, perhaps, or possibly a visit to a well-loved grandmother who always smelled of lavender water.

For those who prefer scientific evidence for the effects of essential oils on the mind, let me draw your attention to some experiments carried out by John Steele (an American research worker) and Maxwell Cade, a British biophysicist. Volunteers were wired up to an ECG (electro-encephalogram) machine called a 'Mind Mirror' (developed by Geoffrey Blundell in 1978) which records brainwave patterns. They observed the effects on the mind of inhaling various essential oils on cotton wool. Those oils which are known to stimulate clarity of thought (rosemary, basil or peppermint) produced more beta brainwaves indicating a state of alertness. Some of the floral antidepressants, such as neroli and jasmine, induced more alpha, theta and delta waves, indicating a quietening of mental 'chatter' and the mind moving into a state approaching meditation.

Critics of aromatherapy have pointed out that the sense of smell becomes quickly exhausted as the olfactory cells in the nose soon become saturated and cease to detect the aroma, so the effects of aromatherapy can only be short-lived. But, as Marguerite Maury and other eminent people in the field of aromatherapy have discovered, the effects can last for some time afterwards, whether the aroma is still perceptible or not.

This may also have much to do with the fact that aromatic molecules, when inhaled, reach the lungs and diffuse from the air sacs into the surrounding blood capillaries. From here they are carried in the blood and exert a physical effect very similar to that of herbal medicine.

The detrimental effects of some odours (such as toxic industrial chemicals) and the results of glue-sniffing on youngsters is proof enough that odours, beneficial or otherwise, do enter the body as gases and can alter the physical and mental health of people and animals too.

PERFUME PREFERENCE

Everyone secretes substances called pheromones which are responsible for their own individual body scent. No two people smell exactly alike, but there are similarities between races, and this may be largely to do with the type of food eaten.

Top perfumer Paul Johnson, an Englishman working for a company in Grasse, France, was baffled for some time by the Scandinavian and Japanese preference for floral perfumes and their shared dislike of animal fixatives such as civet and musk (these are not used in aromatherapy). He came to the conclusion that the greatest similarity between these two geographical areas was their diet of fish.

High dairy food consumers, such as the Dutch, plump for light floral fragrances, whereas mutton and garlic eating Moslems prefer rose perfumes. In the Far East, and in the tropical countries where the diet is high in spices, people prefer the heavy animal-like scents with plenty of fixatives.

Emotions, illness, the pill, and hormonal changes such as pregnancy and the menopause all influence our body odour and our perfume preferences. This helps to explain why we go off certain essential oils, and begin to enjoy the ones previously distasteful to us. As we grow older, our bodies secrete different pheromones, and consequently a favourite perfume from our teens may seem totally obnoxious to us in maturity.

In aromatherapy, the axiom is: always be guided by your own aroma preference. We are instinctively drawn to the fragrance of an oil that is right for our physical and emotional needs at the time.

SKIN ABSORPTION

Many people believe that the skin is an impervious covering, the sole function of which is to keep the blood and organs in and water out. To suggest to them that the skin is capable of absorbing essential oils and diffusing them across the fine capillaries into the main bloodstream is bound to meet with a certain amount of scepticism, if not ridicule.

It is true that water and watery substances cannot be absorbed into the bloodstream through the skin, although the upper layers will *temporarily* hold a little water. This is particularly noticeable after a long soak in the bath, the pads of your fingertips will take on a wrinkled appearance. However, René Gattfossé, the 'father' of modern aromatherapy, established without a doubt that the skin *can* absorb fatty substances provided that their molecular structure is small enough.

Incidentally, the 'black witches' of antiquity used poisonous ointments, impregnated with extract of hemlock and other lethal plants, to see off their enemies. The horrific effect of toxic substances when absorbed through the skin has been witnessed. Even orthodox medics are now using certain drugs, particularly oestrogens, in transcutaneous applications because they are safer and more easily absorbed that way than orally.

The skin is a two-way system, capable of both absorption

and excretion. When we eat spicy or garlicky foods, the odour will be noticeable on our breath; the odoriferous molecules will also be secreted through the pores of the skin with the sweat.

In skin absorption, it is thought that the essential oils, with their very fine molecular structure, pass through the hair follicles, which contain sebum, an oily liquid with which they have an affinity. From here they diffuse into the bloodstream or are taken up by the lymph and interstitial fluid (a liquid surrounding all body cells) to other parts of the body.

If the skin is healthy, it takes only a few minutes for the oil to be absorbed; much longer if the skin is congested or if there is much subcutaneous fat. The skin cannot absorb essential oils when perspiring.

Oils applied to the skin can also affect the underlying organs and nerves that supply them. Various areas of the skin are associated with different spinal nerves. Pain or loss of sensation in a particular area indicates malfunction of an organ or area of the body served by the same nerve. Massage with essential oils over the affected area can thus influence the nerves associated with it. These special areas are called dermatones.

Although essential oils are sometimes administered as internal medicine, they are generally more effective when taken up by the skin. This is also true of evening primrose oil. Although a 'fixed oil' rather than a volatile essence, it appears to work better when applied externally for the treatment of hyperactivity in children. Incidentally, vitamins were applied in this way to treat severely vitamin-deficient ex-prisoners after the Second World War who were too ill to take them by mouth.

ESSENTIAL OILS AND HORMONES

Some essential oils contain plant hormones (phytohormones). Fennel, for example, contains a substance very similar in its chemical structure to oestrogen. It is used in aromatherapy to help those suffering from pre-menstrual syndrome, menopausal difficulties and as an anti-wrinkle skin treatment oil.

However, most essential oils appear to work on the endocrine (hormonal) system indirectly. They can act as triggers to influence hormone secretions of various glands and some of them restore the whole endocrine system to a more balanced state.

It has been known for centuries that plants such as fennel, caraway and fenugreek stimulate the flow of milk, whereas peppermint and sage decrease the flow. Of the many other essential oils known to balance or stimulate hormone secretions, the following are particularly noteworthy.

Garlic helps to balance thyroid secretion.
Basil, geranium, pine and *rosemary* stimulate the adrenal cortex.
Eucalyptus, geranium and *juniper* reduce excessive blood-sugar levels.
Clary sage, lavender and *ylang-ylang* lower high blood pressure.
Camphor and *rosemary* raise low blood pressure.
Lemon and *hyssop* act as regulators of blood pressure; they can raise or lower it.
Cypress balances female sex-hormones, which is particularly useful during the menopause.
Jasmine (an absolute) and *sandalwood* are known to help impotence and frigidity. They are thought to have a hormonal action. Other 'aphrodisiac' oils such as *rose* and *neroli* appear to act more on the emotional level.

Although scientists have tried to duplicate essential oils in the laboratory, they do not have the same beneficial effect. They lack the vital enzymes and probably a multitude of other substances in plants as yet undiscovered. But, above all, they lack the essential 'life-force' found only in nature.

SHELF-LIFE OF ESSENTIAL OILS

Essential oils evaporate readily, and are easily damaged by light, extremes of temperature and prolonged exposure to oxygen in the air. Always buy essences that are sold in well-stoppered, dark glass bottles with an *accurate* dropper cap. There is nothing more infuriating than a fountain of essence when you require only one drop!

Essences, in theory, will keep for years, but the more often you open the bottle the greater the chance of oxidation and a reduction in the oil's therapeutic properties. You can tell when an essence has passed its prime by its cloudy appearance and altered aroma. If stored carefully in a dry dark place away from direct heat, they will keep for at least one year (from one harvest to another) with no problem at all.

Once diluted in vegetable oil for massage, the shelf-life is drastically reduced to about two or three months. Massage oils may keep a little longer with the addition of 5 per cent wheatgerm oil to the vegetable oil base. Wheatgerm oil has anti-oxidant properties as well as being good for stretch marks, ageing skin and scarring.

3

Twenty-five Essential Oils

The essential oils described here are some of the most commonly used in aromatherapy. Although the main therapeutic properties are listed, please refer to Chapter 6 for a more detailed guide to treatment for specific ailments.

Although the emotional effects of essential oils are largely subjective, I have included under each oil in the list a note describing its generally accepted psychotherapeutic effect. However, this information is meant as a rough guide. In my own experience, and this has been confirmed by aroma trials carried out at Warwick University in England, aroma preference is vital. If we dislike the aroma of an essential oil, it is possible to block its effect on the central nervous system.

For those of you who wish to stock up on some basic 'essential essentials', but have no idea where to begin, I have marked with an asterisk those essences which may be most helpful. To these, you may like to include one of the luxury oils such as rose otto or neroli should your finances stretch that far.

Basil	Frankincense	Orange
Bergamot*	Geranium*	Patchouli
Camomile*	Juniper	Peppermint
Cedarwood	Lavender*	Rose otto
Clary sage	Lemon	Rosemary*
Coriander	Marjoram	Sandalwood
Cypress	Myrrh	Tea tree*
Eucalyptus*	Neroli	Ylang-ylang*
Fennel		

BASIL
(Ocimum basilicum)

An annual herb growing to about 3 feet (1 m) high with small yellowish or pinkish flowers. Basil is native to southern Asia and the Middle East, and is now grown mainly as a culinary herb. The essential oil has a faint yellowish tint and is obtained by distillation of the leaves. The aroma is agreeably spicy, vaguely reminiscent of cloves.

Basil is primarily a nerve tonic - it alleviates mental fatigue, anxiety and nervous insomnia. It stimulates the appetite, relieves flatulence and also has an expectorant action. Inhaling the essence can, according to Valnet, restore the sense of smell lost due to chronic catarrh and rhinitis.

Uses: Bronchitis, colds, indigestion, scanty menstrual periods, whooping cough.

Emotional: Sleeplessness due to nervous tensions and anxiety coupled with 'cold' feelings. Hysteria, mental fatigue.

Blends well with: Citrus oils, geranium, neroli.

CAUTION: Avoid during pregnancy or if you have sensitive skin. Use *half* the recommended quantities suggested for other oils (see Chapter 4).

BERGAMOT
(Citrus bergamia)

Bergamot essence is extracted by expression of the skins of the small, greenish citrus fruits grown mainly in Italy for the perfume industry. The essence has the colour of clear emeralds and a delightful scent rather like a blend of oranges and lemons with a slightly spicy overtone. It should not be confused with the garden herb of the same name whose leaves have a similar scent and are used to make oswega tea.

Bergamot is one of the classic ingredients of eau-de-Cologne; it is the flavouring agent of Earl Grey tea and an ingredient of a popular sun-tan cream.

Bergamot reigns supreme as an antidepressant, if its scent is liked, and makes a wonderful bath or massage oil used alone or blended with other essences to uplift depressed spirits.

Uses: Acne, colic, cystitis, fevers, halitosis, indigestion, oily skin, tonsillitis.

Emotional: Depression, nervous tension.

Blends well with: Lavender, geranium, lemon, camomile, neroli, juniper, coriander, cypress, ylang-ylang.

CAUTION: Try to obtain bergamot F.C.F., which is bergaptene-free. Bergaptene may cause skin pigmentation changes when exposed to sunlight. Bergamot should be used in ½-1 per cent concentration (see Chapter 4).

CAMOMILE, ROMAN
(*Anthemis noblis*) (also spelt CHAMOMILE)

CAMOMILE, GERMAN
(*Matricaria chamomilla*)

Although there are several varieties of camomile grown for medicinal purposes, the two most commonly used in aromatherapy are the Roman and German varieties. The essence is distilled from the daisy-like flower heads. Both plants yield an essence containing the blue-coloured, powerful anti-inflammatory agent azulene. German camomile is richer in the substance and can be almost twice as expensive. The former is yellowish with a fine alcohol-like consistency, but it still retains many useful therapeutic properties. German camomile is totally different in appearance, having a thick and creamy consistency and a curious bluish-green tint that gradually alters to greenish-yellow as it ages or upon exposure to the air.

Both camomiles have a very bitter flavour and a sharp scent to match, but the blue essence has a strange, almost salty overtone, not at all like the usual textbook description of its scent as being 'reminiscent of apples'. However, camomile is one of the most useful essential oils in aromatherapy, having a vast range of therapeutic properties. The oil is indicated in all inflammatory conditions and for dull aches and pains (lavender is the best choice for pain that is sharp and piercing). The scent of camomile can be greatly improved by blending with other essences, although some people adore it just as it is.

Uses: Acne, allergies, eczema, anaemia, boils, herpes, colic, colitis, conjunctivitis (*only* the herb tea), indigestion, insomnia, menopausal problems, migraine, neuralgia, period pains, premenstrual syndrome, rheumatism, skin care (particularly dry, sensitive and reddened skin with broken capillaries), stomach cramps, teething pain, toothache, vomiting, wounds.

Emotional: Hysteria, and when anxiety and stress cause a person to be fretful, irritable or nervous.

Blends well with: Bergamot, geranium, lavender, marjoram, lemon, neroli, rose, ylang-ylang.

CAUTION: For sensitive skin and eczema, use ½ per cent concentration (see Chapter 4).

CEDARWOOD
(*Juniperus Virginiana*)

A large coniferous tree native to North America. The oil is distilled from the sawdust and wood shavings saved from the

American cedar mills. The scent is slightly smoky, but distinctly woody - not unlike the aroma of pencils!

A different variety of cedarwood oil (distilled from *Cedrus atlantica* or Atlas cedarwood) was highly prized by the ancient Egyptians and was put to a myriad of uses. As well as being employed in medicine, cosmetics, perfumery and embalming, it was burnt as incense in the temples.

Cedarwood is principally antiseptic and diuretic, and its effect on the central nervous system is sedative.

Uses: Acne, oily skin conditions, scalp disorders, bronchitis, coughs, colds, flu, catarrh, cystitis, cellulite, pre-menstrual syndrome.

Emotional: Anxiety and nervous tension.

Blends well with: Rose, cypress, juniper, neroli, bergamot.

CAUTION: Avoid during pregnancy. If you have sensitive skin, opt for the milder, albeit more tenacious, Atlas cedarwood.

CLARY SAGE
(*Salvia sclarea*)

Clary is one of the sage family. It is a native of Syria, Italy, southern France and Switzerland. The essential oil is clear with a sweet, almost floral quality. It is produced mainly in France and the USSR for the perfume industry. The essence is obtained by steam distillation of the whole plant.

Clary is to be preferred to common sage (*Salvia officinalis*) in aromatherapy for the latter is very toxic if taken in even small doses. Sage essence can bring on a fit in those suffering from epilepsy, as can the oils of hyssop, fennel and wormwood. Clary sage, however, has very similar therapeutic properties to sage, but is non-toxic and has a much sweeter aroma.

Clary is an excellent nerve tonic. It is warming and sedative and is said to induce feelings of comfort and even mild intoxication (euphoria?) in some people, though I have to admit that this has not been my own experience of the essence.

Uses: Absence of menstrual periods, boils, colic, excessive sweating, flatulence, high blood pressure, insect bites and stings, indigestion, leucorrhoea, painful periods, throat infections, thrush, whooping cough.

Emotional: Hysteria or nervous depression which results in sleeplessness.

Blends well with: Cypress, lavender, juniper, citrus oils, geranium.

CAUTION: Avoid during pregnancy.

CORIANDER
(*Coriandrum sativum*)

Coriander is an umbelliferous plant indigenous to southern Europe. It is cultivated practically worldwide, but chiefly in the USSR. Coriander has been used since ancient times as a medicinal and culinary herb and in perfumery. The essence is obtained by steam distillation of the fruit (so-called seeds). It is a fine colourless oil with an agreeable piquant, yet slightly sweet, aroma.

Coriander tea is chiefly used as a medicine to relieve flatulence and stomach cramps. Externally, it may be used in a 2–3 per cent concentration (two or three drops to one tea-spoonful of vegetable oil) as a massage oil for rheumatic pain.

It has a warm, stimulating effect on mind and body and makes a delightful winter bath or massage oil in combination with any of the citrus or spicy essences.

Uses: Colic, flatulence, loss of appetite, nervous dyspepsia, rheumatic pains.

Emotional: Formerly held to be an aphrodisiac. The oil used in baths, massage or inhalation will help nervous debility. It will aid a flagging memory due to boredom or lack of stimulation.

Blends well with: Bergamot, lemon, neroli, orange, cypress and all the spices.

CYPRESS
(*Cupressus sempervirens*)

A tall conical-shaped tree of the conifer family, indigenous to the East and the Mediterranean countries. The tree has figured largely in the medicine of the ancients, notably the Egyptians, Assyrians and the Greeks.

The essential oil is obtained by steam distillation of the leaves and the fruits (cones). It has a dry, refreshing, almost smoky quality. Its effects on the body are similar to those of witch hazel - primarily astringent, and therefore valuable where there is excess loss of fluid (excessive perspiration, heavy menstrual loss). The latter effect on the menstrual cycle may be due to a plant hormone (phytohormone) with the ability to normalise female sex hormones, particularly when related to the menopause. Cypress is helpful blended with clary sage and used in baths and massage for hot flushes.

Cypress may be regarded as a specific for the treatment of piles and varicose veins (with diet and life-style adaptations). Its astringent properties have a locally constricting action on the veins.

Cypress makes a refreshing, yet sedative, bath oil and is particularly good in the summer, perhaps blended with lemon.

Uses: Diarrhoea, haemorrhage (local), incontinence, influenza, loss of voice, menopausal problems, painful periods, piles, pyrrhoea of the gums, rheumatism, skin care (oily skin conditions), spasmodic coughs, varicose veins, whooping cough.

Emotional: Its sedative action will help those suffering from nervous tension.

Blends well with: Clary sage, citrus oils, lavender, marjoram.

EUCALYPTUS
(Eucalyptus globulus)

The eucalyptus tree is known also as the gum-tree. There are over 300 species, some reaching a height of 480 feet (145m). The tree is indigenous to Australia but about 50 species may be found in the Mediterranean countries. The essence is clear with a camphoraceous aroma and is obtained by steam distillation of the leaves.

Eucalyptus reigns supreme in feverish conditions of the respiratory tract such as colds and 'flu. It is familiar to most of us as an inhalant, chest rub or a cough sweet ingredient. It has a pronounced cooling effect on the body, and, according to Valnet, marked anti-viral properties.

As well as being one of the best antiseptics for cuts and wounds, the oil has a diuretic and antiseptic effect on the urinary tract and is valuable in cystitis.

One interesting property of eucalyptus, in common with geranium and juniper, is its ability to lower excessive blood-sugar levels, and therefore it is helpful to diabetics.

Eucalyptus has a predominantly stimulating effect on the nervous system, and, in theory, should help those suffering from lethargic states of mind and body.

Uses: Bronchitis, burns, catarrh, colds, coughs, cystitis, diabetes, diarrhoea, fevers, herpes, influenza, leucorrhoea, measles, migraine, neuralgia, rheumatism, scarlet fever, sinusitis, throat infections, ulcers of the skin, wounds.

Blends well with: Lemon, lemon grass, melissa, lavender, pine, cypress, juniper, tea tree.

FENNEL, SWEET
(*Foeniculum vulgare var. dulcis*)

A member of the umbellifarac family which includes aniseed, caraway and coriander. It is indigenous to the Mediterranean and the Middle East. The plant grows to about 5 feet (1.5m) with bright golden flowers. The essence obtained by distillation of the fruit is clear, with an aniseed aroma.

Fennel exerts a disinfectant and anti-inflammatory action on the respiratory and digestive organs. It has a certain anti-toxic effect and can be useful to counteract the build-up of toxins in the body in such conditions as gout and cellulite (a build-up of fluid and toxic waste in the fatty layers under the skin). It can also be effective in some cases of obesity and has been used for such for hundreds of years. It may be due to its diuretic action.

For thousands of years fennel has been used to stimulate the flow of milk.

Uses: Absence of periods outside pregnancy, bruises, cellulite, colic, constipation, flatulence, gout, indigestion, insufficient milk, irregular periods, loss of appetite, nausea, obesity, pyrrhoea of the gums, respiratory infections, retention of urine, urinary infections.
Blends well with: Lemon, sandalwood, lavender, geranium.

CAUTION: To be avoided during the first trimester of pregnancy. It should also be avoided if you suffer from epilepsy; it may trigger a fit if used in high concentrations. Always use the lowest quantities of this oil, as it may irritate the skin (see Chapter 4).

FRANKINCENSE
(*Boswellia carteri*)(also known as OLIBANUM)

The essential oil of frankincense is extracted from the gum exuded from a small North African tree. It was highly prized in the ancient world, and, along with myrrh, was one of the first gum incenses to be burnt in the temples of ancient Egypt. The essence is yellowish with an interesting balsamic, slightly spicy aroma.

Frankincense is a valuable oil for its effects on the mind. The penetrating aroma and its ability to deepen the breathing make it a helpful aid in meditation. It helps one to see which path to take and therefore is useful in the type of depression where a person is confused and needs to get moving.

Frankincense is also used in aromatherapy for skin care and respiratory infections.

Uses: Bronchitis, catarrh, coughs, laryngitis, leucorrhoea, meditation aid, skin care (particularly dull, wrinkled or ageing skin), wounds.

Emotional: Indecision and fear of the future. Dwelling on unpleasant past events.

Blends well with: Cedarwood, lavender, myrrh, neroli, rose, sandalwood, orange, lemon, and all the spices.

GERANIUM
(*Pelargonium graveolens*)

The plant is indigenous to Algeria, Réunion, Madagascar and Guinea. Essence of Geranium is distilled from the whole plant. It is clear or faintly green with a sweet, refreshing scent. Its effect on the body is primarily balancing.

The oil is tonic and cleansing to both liver and kidneys and is indicated wherever there is poor elimination generally.

Blended with rosemary in a massage oil, it is valuable as an external treatment for areas of fluid retention, puffy ankles for example, or used alone in baths and massage oil for premenstrual fluid retention. Geranium has a stimulating effect on the lymphatic system and will help to drain excess fluid and toxic waste through the lymph ducts.

Geranium is an adrenal cortex stimulant, and so has a balancing effect on hormone production. It is a valuable oil during the menopause and also for pre-menstrual tension.

Geranium's balancing effect can be used to normalize the skin's sebum secretion (oil balance) and so can be used for excessively oily or dry skin conditions. It is mildly astringent, soothing and healing and can be used as a substitute for rose in skin care where the cost of that oil would be prohibitive.

In common with eucalyptus and juniper, geranium has the ability to lower excessive blood-sugar levels, and therefore, is helpful to those suffering from diabetes.

My dentist uses geranium essence as a healing antiseptic after removing a nerve from a tooth. Unfortunately, the use of essential oils in dentistry has seen a marked decline in favour of synthetic substitutes.

Uses: Burns, diabetes, eczema (dry), fluid retention, premenstrual syndrome, gum infections, lice, menopausal problems, mouth ulcers, neuralgia, ringworm, shingles, skin care, sore throats, tonsillitis, thrush, wounds.

Emotional: Geranium has uplifting effects very similar to bergamot. It balances those whose minds are constantly in a whirl. But used in too-high concentrations, or on people who are already calm by nature, it can have a stimulating effect.

Blends well with: Most other essences, particularly with bergamot, neroli, lemon, lavender and juniper.

CAUTION: If you have sensitive skin, use in a low concentration (see Chapter 4) or avoid altogether.

JUNIPER
(*Juniperus communis*)

An evergreen shrub indigenous to the northern hemisphere. The essence is obtained by steam distillation of the berries. It is clear or yellowish green with an aroma similar to that of cypress but somehow more piercing, almost peppery.

Juniper is tonic and stimulating. It will help the body to rid itself of accumulated toxic wastes such as uric acid in rheumatism and arthritis. Used externally it will give relief from the pain of these conditions. As an inhalation, juniper is valuable for respiratory infections such as coughs, colds and 'flu.

In skin care, the oil in a low concentration of ½ per cent (one drop to two teaspoonfuls of vegetable oil) will help 'weepy' eczema and acne.

Uses: Absence of periods outside pregnancy, acne, arthritis, coughs, cystitis, dermatitis, eczema (wet), fumigation, gout, leucorrhoea, piles, respiratory infections, rheumatism, skin care, urinary tract infections, fluid retention.

Emotional: A juniper bath will help to shake off nervous tension brought on by absorbing the negative emotions of others.

Blends well with: Citrus oils, lavender, rosemary, geranium, sandalwood, cedarwood.

CAUTION: To be avoided during pregnancy.

LAVENDER
(*Lavendula officinalis*, *L. augustifolia* or *L. vera*)

Lavender originated in the mountainous regions of the Mediterranean. The Romans used it to add to their bath water and the English name came from the latin *lavare*, 'to wash'.

English lavender is often regarded as the finest in the world, and vast quantities of lavender oil are produced in France for the perfume industry.

The best essence is distilled from the flowering tops (it is present in the leaves as well) and has a faintly yellow tint and the familiar refreshing scent that hardly needs description. Spike lavender (*Lavendula spica latifolia*) has a camphorated aroma and is the most useful of the lavenders for respiratory disorders.

Lavender is regarded amongst aromatherapists as the most versatile essential oil at their disposal. It has a myriad of uses, but it reigns supreme in skin conditions (particularly acne and burns) and is a superb sedative and pain-killing essence. Its effect on body and mind is primarily balancing. It blends well with almost all other essences, including frankincense and myrrh.

Uses: Abscess, acne, asthma, boils, bronchitis, burns, catarrh, colds, coughs, cuts, cystitis, dermatitis, earache, eczema, fainting, flatulence, high blood pressure, infectious illness, insect bites and stings, leucorrhoea, laryngitis, migraine, muscular aches and pains, psoriasis, periods (scanty and painful), pre-menstrual syndrome, perfuming rooms and as an air freshener, sinusitis, skin care (all skin types), sciatica, worms.

Emotional: Its balancing action is best suited to those suffering from hysterical states of mind or wildly fluctuating moods. Also for insomnia, nervous tension and other forms of depression.

Blends well with: Almost all other essences, but particularly with bergamot, geranium, marjoram, camomile, clary sage, neroli, rosemary, ylang-ylang.

LEMON
(*Citrus limonum*)

Essence of lemon is produced mainly in Spain and Portugal, and is obtained simply by expression of the outer rind of the fruit.

As a bath oil, lemon is tonic and invigorating. It is neither too sedative nor too stimulating and blends well with many other essences. Lemon will sharpen the sweet and cloying (ylang-ylang), 'masculinise' the feminine (rose, lavender), 'lift' the heavy lingerers (sandalwood, frankincense), or will simply add a cheerful and familiar note to blends.

Uses: Acidity (stomach), arthritis, anaemia, coughs, cuts (it arrests bleeding), insect bites and stings (neat), loss of appetite, rheumatism, sore throats, verrucae and warts.

Emotional: Feelings of lethargy or congestion of mind and body.

Blends well with: Most essences, but particularly with camomile, ylang-ylang, fennel, frankincense, lavender, geranium, eucalyptus, juniper.

CAUTION: Citrus essences may cause skin pigmentation changes when exposed to sunlight.

MARJORAM, Sweet
(Origanum majorana)

An aromatic herb indigenous to the Far East and the Mediterranean. It is not an annual, but is treated as such in temperate climates for it will not withstand cold winters. The essential oil is obtained by steam distillation of the flowering tops; it has a yellowish tint and an agreeable spicy aroma very similar to coriander, but it lacks the lighter, fruitier qualities of that oil.

Marjoram is predominantly warming to body and mind and is indicated for the treatment of 'cold' conditions such as bronchitis, rheumatism, grief and loneliness. Marjoram is a reputed anaphrodisiac (diminishes sexual desire) and was said to have been used in the past to quell the sexual desire of the inmates of orphanages and monasteries. However, some herbals suggest that marjoram has the opposite effect! It may be safe to assume that the herb's effect varies from one person to another. After all, we each respond differently to the foods that we eat and the dosage of medicines. Incidentally, too much of a herb or essential oil very often has the opposite effect to that expected.

When massaged into the abdomen (in a clockwise rotation) marjoram will soothe a colicky stomach and intestinal pain. It is also one of the most effective oils for the treatment of menstrual cramps – use in a compress.

Uses: Arthritis, bronchitis, bruises, colds, constipation, flatulence, headache, high blood pressure, indigestion, leucorrhoea, migraine, painful periods.

Emotional: Grief and loneliness, insomnia, hysteria and nervous tension.

Blends well with: Lavender, bergamot, camomile, cypress.

CAUTION: Avoid during pregnancy.

MYRRH
(Commiphora myrrha)

The essential oil of myrrh is extracted from the gum of the myrrh bush, native of north-east Africa and of the same botanical family as frankincense. The essence is reddish-brown with the consistency of treacle and consequently difficult to use unless gently heated. Its aroma is not appealing to most people, having a dry, balsamic quality, but gives an interesting earthy quality to blends if used in small quantities.

Myrrh, like frankincense, was highly prized in the ancient world for medicine, incense, perfumery and embalming. It has powerful anti-inflammatory properties and can be used to treat 'weepy' wounds.

It is one of the best treatments for mouth ulcers and vaginal thrush (see Chapter 5).

Uses: Absence of periods outside pregnancy, catarrh, coughs, diarrhoea, flatulence, gingivitis, leucorrhoea, mouth infections, pyrrhoea, piles, thrush, ulcers (mouth and skin), wounds.

Emotional: Coldness.

Blends well with: Frankincense, sandalwood, cedarwood, patchouli.

CAUTION: Avoid during pregnancy.

NEROLI, Orange Blossom
(Citrus bigaradia, C. vulgaris and *C. aurantium)*

The best quality essence is distilled from the blossom of the bitter orange tree (*Citrus bigaradia*). It has a yellowish tint and a sweetish, yet dry, scent – not at all citrusy. Orange flower water is obtained during the distillation process of the oil. Much of the essential oil is produced in France and Italy for the perfume industry. It is one of the principal ingredients of the best quality eau-de-Cologne. Neroli, like rose otto, is one of the most expensive essential oils.

It is one of the best anti-depressant, sedative oils, having a slightly hypnotic effect. It induces sleep, alleviates nervous tension and is another of the oils credited as an aphrodisiac.

Neroli has the ability to stimulate the growth of healthy new skin cells and was used by Marguerite Maury in her skin-rejuvenating treatments for her wealthy, middle-aged clients. She also credited lavender with this property. Neroli may be used as a facial oil for most skin types, but particularly for dry or sensitive skins. For the latter, always use the lowest concentration (one drop to two or even three teaspoons of vegetable oil).

Uses: Chronic diarrhoea, palpitations, skin care.

Emotional: Depression, particularly of a nervous or hysterical nature. It will help to alleviate insomnia and is a good remedy for shock.

Blends well with: Camomile, coriander, geranium, jasmine, lavender, citrus oils, rose, ylang-ylang.

ORANGE, BITTER
(Citrus vulgaris)

ORANGE, SWEET
(Citrus aurantium)

(Oil of mandarin has similar properties but is much milder and can be safely used for children externally in ½–1 per cent dilution.)

The orange tree yields three different essential oils: orange (from the fruit); petit grain (from the leaves and young shoots); and neroli (from the flowers).

The essence of bitter orange, known also as Oil of Bigarade, and sweet orange essence, Oil of Portugal, is obtained from the outer skins of the fruit by simple pressure. The oil is fine and almost watery in consistency with a yellow tint. It is used widely in the food and pharmaceutical industries as a flavouring agent, but it has therapeutic properties of its own. It may be used in steam inhalations for chronic bronchitis. It will soothe dry, irritated skin but *only* if used in the smallest quantities –

one drop to three teaspoons of vegetable oil.

Orange oil adds a warm and comforting, yet jolly note to bath oil blends, massage oils, perfumes and room sprays.

Uses: Bronchitis, chills, colds, skin care.

Emotional: A need for frivolity and warmth.

Blends well with: Coriander (and all the spices), cypress, frankincense, juniper.

CAUTION: Citrus oils cause skin pigmentation changes when exposed to sunlight.

PATCHOULI
(Pogostemon patchouli)

A highly odoriferous plant native to India. The oil is obtained by distillation of the dried leaves; it is dark amber with an extremely tenacious aroma which you will either love or detest. The odour is earthy, some might say musty, yet it becomes much more pleasant once the sour element has had time to wear off. The oil has been used for thousands of years in India for medicinal purposes, but chiefly as an aphrodisiac and to perfume cloth. Patchouli is also one of the few oils that actually improves with age: a twenty-year-old essence will be extremely mellow and fragrant.

Patchouli is primarily antiseptic, antibiotic, anti-fungal and fortifying, therefore it should be helpful in infectious illness and for fungal infections such as ringworm and athlete's foot. However, aromatherapists tend to use the oil to help oily skin conditions; to stimulate the growth of healthy hair; to combat cellulite and, if the aroma is liked, to heal distressing emotions. Although patchouli is generally regarded as a sedative oil, I have known it to have an energizing effect on some people.

Uses: Acne, oily skin, scalp disorders, cracked skin, fluid retention, cellulite, pre-menstrual syndrome.

Emotional: Anxiety and depression.

Blends well with: Rose, bergamot, geranium, lavender, pine needle, myrrh, ginger, ylang-ylang.

PEPPERMINT
(Mentha piperita)

Oil of peppermint is a fine colourless essence obtained by distillation of the flowering plant. Although native to Europe, much of the world's supply of peppermint, and its essential oil, is produced in the U.S.A. Peppermint oil is widely used in the food and pharmaceutical industries as a flavouring agent, but it has a multitude of therapeutic properties. The oil can be used in inhalations for headaches and sinusitis. Many text books on aromatherapy advocate the use of peppermint for irritated skin conditions, but I feel this should be avoided by the lay-person as the oil can be extremely irritant to the skin if used in concentrations above ½-per cent. If you wish to use it as a bath oil, first dilute as little as two or three drops in some vegetable oil before adding to the water. It is better to use the lowest concentration and top it up with three or four drops of another essential oil to enhance the aroma.

Peppermint is a stimulant and is best used during the day rather than just before bedtime – unless you are feeling extremely uncomfortable and 'blocked up' with a bad cold and would be unable to sleep anyway.

In many cases, peppermint is best suited to conditions of an acute or short-term nature. Digestive upsets of a chronic or more generalised nature, for example, may respond best to camomile.

Peppermint has 'cephalic' properties: it is reputed to stimulate the brain, aiding clarity of thought (rosemary and basil are two others). If you are about to sit an exam or face a similar ordeal, especially if you have a head cold, sprinkle a few drops of peppermint oil onto a handkerchief and inhale whenever you wish.

Uses: Bronchitis, colds, colic, coughs (dry), diarrhoea, fainting, fevers, 'flu, halitosis, headache, indigestion, insect repellant, migraine, nausea, scabies, sinusitis, travel sickness, vomiting.

Emotional: Sudden shock, mental fatigue, inability to think clearly.

Blends well with: The essence tends to overpower blends, but if used in tiny amounts it may be acceptable with larger proportions of one of the following: lavender, marjoram, rosemary.

CAUTION: Avoid during the first trimester of pregnancy.

ROSE OTTO
(Rosa damascena)

Rose essence is obtained by distillation of the flower petals. Although there are thousands of varieties of rose in a multitude of colours, the variety used for this essence is ruby-red and grows in Bulgaria. The oil is almost colourless and is semi-solid at room temperature. The aroma is truly exquisite (to my nose at any rate!), very mellow with a hint of vanilla and cloves. It is quite different from the less costly rose absolute, which is extracted by solvents and is yellow-orange rather than clear.

Rosewater is a useful by-product of the distillation process and can be used as an eyewash for inflammation of the eyelids, or a skin tonic for even the most delicate of complexions.

In aromatherapy, rose otto is generally used in skin care and for healing distressing emotions. It is a superb anti-depressant and a reputed aphrodisiac. The oil is especially indicated for 'female complaints' - heavy or irregular periods, for example. The action of rose on the uterus is cleansing and tonic.

Rose otto also makes an excellent facial oil for all skin types, but especially for dry, ageing and sensitive skins. The oil has a tonic effect on the capillaries and can be used to treat and prevent thread veins.

Rose otto is so highly concentrated that a tiny amount will be effective - one drop will perfume 25ml of vegetable oil, for example, or a bath full of warm water.

Uses: Conjunctivitis (use only the rosewater), constipation, hangover (rose has a cleansing effect on the liver), headaches, heavy or irregular periods, leucorrhoea, pre-menstrual syndrome, nausea, skin care, uterine disorders, vomiting.

Emotional: Depression, grief, nervous tension.

Blends well with: Most essences, especially patchouli, cedarwood, bergamot, sandalwood, camomile, ylang-ylang.

ROSEMARY
(*Rosmarinus officinalis*)

An evergreen shrub indigenous to the Mediterranean coast, but now widely cultivated for ornamental, culinary, medicinal and perfumery purposes. Most of the supplies used commercially are imported from France, Spain and Morocco. The essential oil, obtained by steam distillation of the whole plant, is clear with a camphoraceous aroma.

Rosemary is one of the three cephalic oils (the others are basil and peppermint); it stimulates the brain, aiding clarity of thought and the memory. It also alleviates fatigue. The piercing aroma of rosemary makes it a beneficial steam inhalation for many respiratory disorders such as bronchitis, colds and 'flu.

Rosemary is anti-rheumatic and can be used in baths, compresses and massage oils for both rheumatism and arthritis.

For centuries rosemary has been a renowned skin and hair tonic. It will eliminate dandruff, stimulate hair growth and enhance the colour of dark hair. It may be used as an aromatic water or facial oil for most skin types, particularly dingy city skins inclined to be oily.

Uses: Arthritis, bronchitis, burns, colds, dandruff, dyspepsia, flatulence, gout, headache, high cholesterol, low blood pressure, influenza, migraine, palpitations, rheumatism, skin care, wounds.

Emotional: Nervous debility affecting the memory and clarity of thought.

Blends well with: Basil, bergamot, peppermint, lavender, juniper.

CAUTION: Avoid during the first trimester of pregnancy.

SANDALWOOD
(*Santalum album*)

A small, parasitic tree (it buries its roots in those of neighbouring trees) growing to a height of 20-30 feet (6-9m). Sandalwood is native to the East Indies, the best quality oil coming from Mysore.

Sandalwood has been used since antiquity in medicine, perfumery, incense and embalming. The essence is obtained from the heart wood of the tree by a method of steam distillation. It is a clear, or faintly greenish, viscid essence with a sweet, smooth aroma. Its scent cannot be fully experienced until applied to the skin. However, sandalwood has the curious ability to be completely undetectable to a few individuals, yet incredibly persistent to others!

The three main areas of its use are in skin care (dry, ageing skin types), respiratory disorders and emotional disturbance. Sandalwood essence is both a sedative and a pulmonary antiseptic helping to clear catarrh. The aphrodisiac effect of the oil has been renowned since time immemorial. With this, and the combination of its sedative and anti-depressant effects, sandalwood is valuable for the treatment of impotence and frigidity.

Uses: Acne, bronchitis, catarrh, coughs, cystitis, diarrhoea, laryngitis, room perfuming, skin care, vomiting.

Emotional: Depression leading to sexual difficulties, nervous tension, insomnia.

Blends well with: Fennel, frankincense, jasmine, lemon, myrrh, rose, ylang-ylang.

TEA TREE
(*Melaleuca alternifolia*)

An extremely hardy tree native to Australia. It has amazing powers of regeneration; when cut down it will quickly grow again from its original stump. The oil is obtained by distillation of the leaves and twigs. The aroma is somehow reminiscent of a mixture of juniper and cypress, but perhaps less refined, having a strong medicinal overtone. In fact, it is one of the most powerful antiseptic, antiviral and anti-fungal oils available. Like the vigorous habit of the tree itself, the oil is a wonderful immune system stimulant. It reigns supreme where there is infectious illness or debility. Indeed, it has even been successfully employed in Australia to treat AIDS sufferers. More humbly, the oil can be used neat as an antiseptic for wounds.

Uses: Acne, athlete's foot, mouth ulcers, thrush, warts, cold sores, insect bites and stings, coughs, colds, flu, scalp disorders, wounds.

Emotional: In Australia, the oil has been used for years as a standby for treating shock and hysteria – put a few drops in the bath.

Blends well with: Does not blend very well with other oils, but the aroma can be improved by mixing with lemon, lavender or pine.

YLANG-YLANG
(*Cananga odorata var. genuina*)

Its name means 'flower of flowers' and it is the blossom of a tree native to the Far East – Java, Sumatra and the Philippines. The essence is obtained by distillation of the flowers and has a yellowish tint. Its aroma is best described as reminiscent of the night-scented stock (*Matthiola bicornis*) with a hint of almond essence. One either adores the oil or dislikes it intensely! Those of the latter category may prefer the oil in its diluted state (one or two drops to two teaspoons of vegetable oil). In this strength, many people find the oil quite exquisite.

Ylang-ylang is primarily sedative; it helps to lower high blood pressure and rapid heart beat (tachycardia) and is credited with aphrodisiac properties.

As a facial oil, it has a soothing effect and is particularly good for oily skin.

Uses: High blood pressure, palpitations, skin care, pre-menstrual syndrome.

Emotional: It has anti-depressant properties particularly suited to those who feel frustrated and angry. It may also be used to help nervous tension, insomnia, frigidity and impotence.

Blends well with: Geranium, lavender, citrus oils, neroli, patchouli, rose.

4

Using Essential Oils

There are a number of ways of using essential oils. They can be added to your bath, made into skin oils, used in steam inhalations for colds and 'flu, as perfumes to subtly influence your mood, and in many other ways to improve your health and vitality. For hints on blending for therapeutic purposes, see Chapter 5.

Let us first turn to the commonest, and perhaps most people the best-known, use - massage.

MASSAGE

There is no denying that a good aromatherapy massage is a truly divine experience; and giving massage can be enjoyable too. You can, of course, massage the oils into your own skin and derive benefit from them, but the most pleasurable and certainly the most relaxing way is to receive massage from a friend.

The very basic massage strokes outlined here are meant only as a guide to enable you to develop your own intuitive style. To learn massage from a book is not easy; you will eventually feel the need to attend a weekend workshop or you may even wish to embark on an extended study course. Having said this, many people are superb intuitive massage therapists and no amount of formal training will improve on their special 'touch'.

The main advantage of serious tuition is that you will be given a good grounding in anatomy and physiology. This will enable you to understand when there is a departure from the normal state; why pain may be occurring in a particular area and when to refer the person to an osteopath, chiropractor or even a surgeon.

The Effects of Massage

Massage will aid the elimination of toxic wastes by stimulating blood circulation and lymphatic drainage. This helps to relieve muscular pain by increasing nutrition to the painful areas and at the same time removing the stagnant toxic wastes such as lactic and carbonic acids which build up in the muscle fibres.

A gruesome experiment was carried out in the nineteenth century to demonstrate the effects of massage on waste disposal. Ink was injected into the leg muscles of two unfortunate rabbits. The leg of one rabbit was massaged regularly. After about a month, the creatures were killed and dissected. Ink was found in the muscles surrounding the injection site of the rabbit that had not been massaged; no trace of ink was found anywhere in the body of the other.

As mind and body are interrelated, the emotional aspect of aromatherapy massage should not be overlooked. When body tension is released, negative emotions such as fear, anxiety, anger, and so forth, begin to melt away. You may feel deeply relaxed and peaceful afterwards or perhaps exhilarated and more energetic than before. The effect will always be balancing: it will calm where there is restlessness or stimulate where there is lethargy.

By combining the power of human touch with the subtle energies of plant essences, we can influence the person on many different levels simultaneously.

When Not To Massage

Massage is contra-indicated in the following conditions: fever, inflammation (of skin and joints), cardiovascular disease, skin rashes or eruptions, swellings, bruises, sprains, torn muscles and ligaments, broken bones, burns and varicose veins. In short, if it hurts, abandon the movement and move on to another area of the body. It is also generally believed that people suffering from cancer should not be massaged because cancer cells may start to spread via the lymphatic system. However, recent evidence does not appear to bear this out. Very gentle aromatherapy massage is being used in many British NHS hospitals to help uplift the spirits of cancer patients.

Before You Begin

The area where you intend to give massage should be aesthetically pleasing and softly lit. Work in natural daylight if possible or under soft lamp or candlelight. Harsh overheated lighting will only serve to remind your subject of an operating table or a visit to the dentist!

Ensure that the room is very warm and draught-free; chilled muscles contract, causing a release of adrenalin – something you are trying to soothe away in the first place.

If you wish to enhance the atmosphere with music, be sure to play that which is specially composed for relaxation. Ordinary music is too jarring; constantly changing in tempo. You will find yourself moving in time to the musical rhythm instead of concentrating on the massage rhythm inherent within you. Massage music should be soft and monotonous; purely background sound. You will find many superb pieces of music specially composed for massage and relaxation at good record shops.

The easiest place to give massage is on a purpose-built couch. But of course many of you will have to work on the floor. Resist the temptation to massage on a bed. Not only will this add enormous strain on your back; the mattress will absorb all the necessary pressure intended for the body. A sleeping bag, strip of foam rubber, thick blankets, a soft rug or a duvet will provide padding under your subject. Cover this with a sheet or towel. Both are easily cleaned should any oil staining occur.

A second sheet or thick towel is needed to cover the areas of the body you are not working on.

Massage Oils

Before choosing an essential oil for massage, or for any other treatment, first read the basic guidelines at the beginning of Chapter 5. It is important to use the correct essential oil, or blend of essences, to suit the physical and emotional needs of the recipient.

Essential oils intended for massage need to be diluted in a natural base oil such as almond, sunflower seed, peach or apricot kernel – cold-pressed or unrefined if possible. These oils are health treatments in themselves; they are rich in fat-soluble nutrients that can easily be absorbed by the skin. Avoid mineral oil (baby oil) because it may clog the pores and even rob the body of some of its fat-soluble nutrients. Good quality vegetable oils are now widely available from health shops and supermarkets.

Essential oils need to be diluted at a rate of ½ to 3 per cent, depending on the person's skin, the strength of the essential oil and the condition for which it is being applied. Lowest concentrations (½ to 1 per cent) are best for facial oils, children, and for anyone with sensitive skin. If your skin is sensitive, it is best to start with the ½ per cent concentration and, if this causes no irritation, increase to 1 per cent, then to 2 per cent if desired. However, a few oils are very strong and should always be used in concentrations no greater than ½ to 1 per cent. These include camomile, basil, lemon grass, ginger, fennel and melissa. I tend also to be wary of oils such as ylang-ylang, black pepper, citrus oils and geranium. These are best used at a concentration no greater than 2 per cent.

Simple Measures

If you intend to mix only enough oil for a single massage, use a 5 ml plastic medicine spoon (available from chemists) to measure the carrier oil. Ordinary teaspoons generally hold less than 5 ml.

Low concentrations for facial oils, children and for those with sensitive skin: For a ½ per cent concentration add *one* drop of essential oil to every *two* 5 ml teaspoonsful of carrier oil. For a 1 or 2 per cent concentration, add one or two drops of essential oil to each 5 ml teaspoonful of carrier oil.

Medium to high concentrations for body oils: For a 2 or 3 per cent concentration, add two or three drops of essential oil to each 5 ml teaspoonful of carrier oil.

For larger quantities of massage oil to be stored in dark glass bottles, fill a 50 ml bottle with carrier oil, then add the required amount of essential oil. For a ½ per cent concentration, add five drops to 50 ml of carrier oil. For a 1 per cent concentration in the same amount of carrier oil, add ten drops of essential oil; for a 2 per cent concentration, add twenty drops and for 3 per cent, add thirty drops. Store in a cool place, and use within two to three months.

Dark glass bottles are generally available from chemists, otherwise recycle any suitable dark glass bottle with a screw cap. The capacity in mls is usually imprinted into the glass at the base of the bottle.

Giving Massage

It would be impossible to describe full-body massage adequately in a book of this size; so I will concentrate on the most important areas in aromatherapy massage – the back, head, face and neck.

Before you begin it is important to remember that, once you have made contact with your subject's body, you should try not to break it until the end of the massage. When you need to apply more oil, ensure that an elbow or a knee is against his or her body. It can feel quite disconcerting to be left waiting for the next stroke.

THE BACK
The back may be regarded as the gateway to the whole person. The body's main nerves branch out from either side of the spine and supply all the internal organs. By relaxing the back muscles and working on areas of muscle tension, stress levels will be reduced. This leads to improved health and a sense of well-being.

Position your subject on his or her front, head to one side, arms relaxed at the sides or loosely bent with the hands at shoulder level. Some people feel more comfortable with a rolled-up towel or cushion under the chest and ankles. Kneel down to one side of your subject. Before oiling your hands, very gently place one hand on the crown of the head and the other at the base of the spine. Hold them there for a few moments to allow your subject to become accustomed to your touch.

1. Oil your hands; rub them together to warm them and the oil. Place your hands at the base of the back, either side of the spine with your fingers relaxed, pointing towards the head. You should never apply pressure to the spine itself, but the strong muscles either side can take firm pressure. Now slide your hands up the back; move your body from the centre until you reach the neck. Slide the hands firmly across the shoulder and then glide them down. As you reach the waist, pull it up gently and return smoothly to the starting position (see Fig. 1).

   It is important to use the whole of your hand; allow your hands to mould the contours of his or her body as if you were sculpting it out of clay. Repeat these long firm strokes several times until the whole of the back is well oiled, but not too slippery. You will find that two to four teaspoonfuls

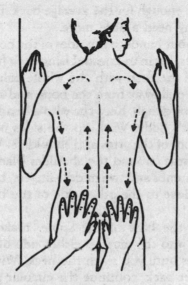

Fig. 1 Long smooth strokes.

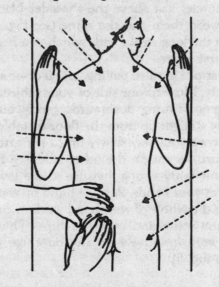

Fig. 2 Kneading.

of oil will be enough for the average back. People with very dry skin may need a little more.

2. Now move your hands to the sides of the body and, starting from the hips, begin to knead. Using each hand alternately, take hold of the flesh with the whole palm of your hand and fingers, pull away from the bone and squeeze as if you were kneading dough. Keep the whole hand in contact with the recipient's body. Work up the sides of the torso and across the tops of the arms and shoulders. When you come to smaller areas (around the shoulder blades for instance) change to thumbs and two middle fingers, but do not pinch the flesh. Move to the other side of the body and repeat (see Fig. 2).

3. Starting at the base of the spine, make small circular movements into the muscles either side of the spine with your thumbs until you reach the neck. With your thumbs on the upper back, continue the circular movements. Do not press on the spine or the shoulder blade itself. Work on the muscles just above the shoulder blades and those lying between them and the spine (see Fig. 3).

4. Return to the long stroke with which you began in Step 1. Repeat three times.

5. The next stroke is called pulling, and is done along the sides of the body. Move to one side of your subject's back. With your fingers pointing downwards gently pull each hand alternately straight up from the floor or table. Start at the hip and work your way slowly up to the armpit and back down again. Repeat on the other side (see Fig. 4).

6. Apply some fairly strong pressure to the lower back with the heels of your hands. Put one hand on top of the other, and using the whole of your hand work in circles from the base of the spine and over the hips. Then using your thumbs, work intuitively on any tightness you may find there (see Fig. 5).

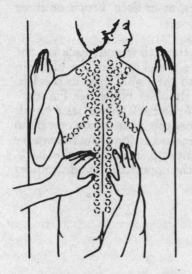

Fig. 3 Thumb circles.

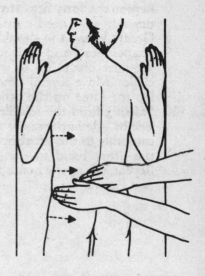

Fig. 4 Pulling.

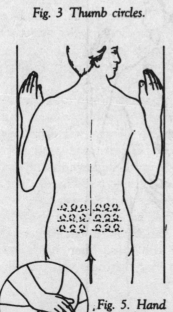

Fig. 5. Hand
-over-hand circles.

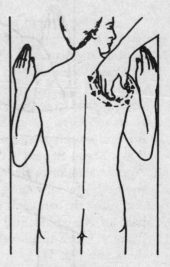

Fig. 6. Rotating skin on the
shoulder blade.

7. Repeat the long firm strokes, as in Step 1, two or three times.
8. Gently knead the shoulders.
9. Shape your hand as if it were a claw and place on the shoulder blade. Try to move the skin over the blade in circles. Move several times to the right, then to the left. Do the same on the other shoulder blade (see Fig. 6).
10. Starting from the middle of the back, place your hands side by side horizontally across the spine. Move one hand smoothly to the left shoulder, and at the same time move the other hand to the right hip, stretching the back. Repeat, taking the hands to the opposite hip and shoulder (see Fig. 7).

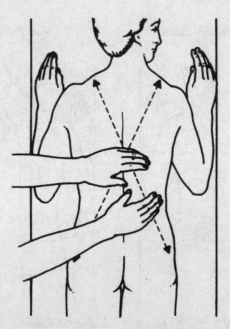

Fig. 7. Stretching the back (1).

11. This time place both your whole forearms horizontally across the back and slide them slowly, yet firmly, apart; one up the back to the top of the shoulders and the other down to the top of the buttocks; use a fair amount of pressure (see Fig. 8).

12. End your massage the same way you began by placing one hand on your subject's head and the other at the base of the spine. When you are ready, move your hands away and cover the person with a towel. Allow him or her to rest for a while to 'come round' in their own time.

This completes the basic back sequence, but add anything you intuitively feel is needed. Work with your whole body, not just your hands and arms. When you are kneading, move gently

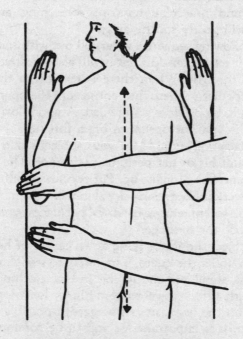

Fig. 8. Stretching the back (2).

from side to side in time with your hands. Keep your movements slow and gently flowing. Allow your natural rhythm to come to the fore. Sensitivity at the outset far outweighs a full routine of complicated strokes if they are carried out in a mechanical and impersonal manner. Most important of all, develop your own unique style.

THE FACE AND HEAD

This is an area of the body quite often neglected in remedial massage therapy, yet a good face and scalp massage can be one of the most uplifting experiences of all time. A violent headache can be safely dissolved within minutes without having to resort to aspirin or paracetamol with their accompanying side-effects. Drugs do nothing to remove the cause of a headache which more often than not stems from nervous and muscular tension; something aromatherapy massage will gently soothe away.

If the following sequence is carried out with sensitivity, not only will it relieve tension but it will also effectively stimulate clarity of thought. When there is tension in the neck and spine, particularly where they connect to the brain at the base of the skull, blood flow is impeded. A good flow of blood to the head is vital for optimum brain function.

Mix a facial oil suitable for your subject's skin type taking into account his or her perfume preference. The skin should be clean and free of make-up. Put two teaspoonfuls of the oil into a saucer; only *extremely* dry skin will need more than this. Ask the person to remove earrings, necklaces or anything that may impede the massage.

Your subject should be lying down on his or her back with a cushion under the knees, if required, to straighten the lower back. The shoulders should be free of clothing, cover the person with a thick towel to keep him or her warm. If you are working on the floor, sit cross-legged if possible or kneel on a cushion. It is important for you to be comfortable as any tension will be perceived by your subject.

THE FACE

1. Before you oil your hands, place them on either side of your subject's head. The heels of your hands should cover the forehead, fingers extending downwards, anchoring the sides of the head. Hold them there for a few moments.
2. Move your hands to the forehead and smoothly stroke the brow, hand-over-hand, up and over the hair to the crown of the head. Repeat several times.
3. Move your hands gently away and dip your fingers into the oil. Rub it into your hands. You will need only a smear of oil for the face; if you drench the skin, oil is liable to seep into the person's eyes.
4. Gently glide your hands over your subject's face starting from the chin, circling the eyes and over the forehead. This is simply to oil the skin before you begin the massage (see Fig. 9).

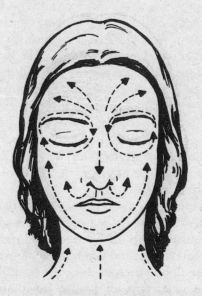

Fig. 9. Oiling the face and neck.

5. Oil your hands a little more generously this time and slide them over the shoulders and up the back of the neck. Go *very* lightly over the throat. Your movements should always be slow and flowing, not brisk and jerky. Use light to medium pressure to avoid dragging the skin, and be particularly careful around the eye area.

6. Place the ball of your thumbs at the centre of the forehead between the eyebrows. Slide both thumbs apart and, when you reach the temples, finish with a little circular flourish before gliding off at the hairline (see Fig. 10).

7. Return to the starting position, but this time a little higher up. Repeat Step 6 and continue, a strip at a time, all the way up the forehead until you reach the hairline (see Fig. 10).

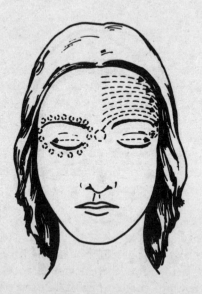

Fig. 10. *Stroking the forehead, pressure points around the eyes, light strokes on the eyelids.*

8. Place your thumbs at the centre between the eyebrows (the 'third eye') and this time slide your thumbs a little more firmly over the brow bone and off the head. Repeat once or twice.

9. Return to the third eye position and this time press your thumbs down quite firmly (your subject will soon tell you if it is too hard) and hold for about three seconds. Lift your thumbs and place them a little further out along the brow bone and repeat the pressure. Repeat this at intervals until you reach the outer corners of the eyes (see Fig. 10).

10. Place your forefinger on the bony ridge *under* the eyes at the inner corners and repeat the pressing movements, a little more lightly this time, until you reach the outer corner. This is helpful to those who suffer from catarrh or sinus congestion.
    CAUTION: Do not apply pressure if the sinuses are swollen and painful (see Fig. 10).

11. Now slide an un-oiled finger or thumb *very lightly* over the eyelids, but not if your subject is wearing contact lenses. Gently rotate the eye itself under the lids, first clockwise then anti-clockwise. Repeat once or twice.

12. Now allow your subject to bathe in darkness for a few moments. Place the heels of your hands gently against both eyes with the fingers extending downwards. Hold them there for up to half a minute if you wish, but no less than ten seconds.

13. Slide your hands to the sides of your subject's head and apply a little pressure to the temples for about ten seconds.

14. Gently stroke the entire face with gentle upward movements as in Step 4.

15. Place the ball of your thumbs at the inner corners of the eyes just below the eye socket. Smooth outwards and upwards towards the temples. Circle the temples as you did in Step 6. Repeat a little lower down, a strip at a time, until you reach the edge of the cheekbone. Repeat the same

movement again just below the bone, pressing lightly upwards (see Fig. 11).

16. Place the forefingers on each side of the nose near the bridge. Using tiny circles, work down the sides of the nose (see Fig. 11).

17. Using your thumbs alternately, stroke down the bridge of the nose from the top to the tip. Circle the tip with the palm of your hand (see Fig. 11).

18. Using your middle fingers, make tiny circles on the cheeks at either side of the nostrils and over the upper lip (see Fig. 11).

19. Place your thumbs on the chin and pull them slowly and firmly outwards and upwards along the jaw bone to the ear.

   Repeat a little further inwards until just below the cheek bone (see Fig. 12).

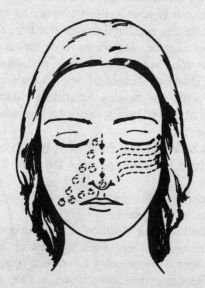

Fig. 11. Stroking and circling the cheeks and nose.

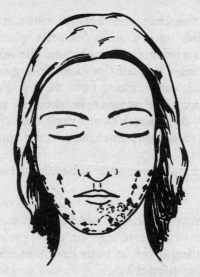

Fig. 12. Stroking and circling the chin and jaw.

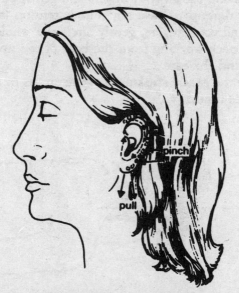

Fig. 13. Working on the ears.

20. Return to the chin and work in tiny circles with your thumbs. Slide your thumbs from the middle of the chin along the jaw bone, finishing behind the ears (see Fig. 12).
21. Work in circles behind the ears. Now gently pinch the edges of each ear, working from the top down to the ear lobes. Repeat once or twice, finishing by pulling the ear lobes gently downwards two or three times. Then with the tips of the forefingers trace around the spiral of the ears (see Fig. 13).
22. Cup your hands over your subject's eyes as in Step 12.

THE NECK
1. Gently turn your subject's head to the left. Place your left hand on his or her forehead; or, if you prefer, support the head by letting it rest in your left hand. Place your right hand on your subject's right shoulder and slide your hand firmly all the way up to the neck. When you reach the base of the skull, use all your fingers and gently circle the area several times to release any muscle tension (see Fig. 14).
2. Using all your fingers, gently circle the whole right side of the neck working from the base of the neck upwards to behind the ears.
3. Repeat the gentle stroking movements, as in Step 2, two or three times.

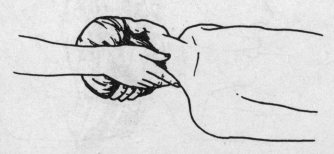

Fig. 14. Stroking and circling the neck.

4. Gently turn your subject's head to the right and repeat Steps 2-3 on the left side.

5. Gently move your subject's head to the middle so that he or she is lying straight once more. Place your hands horizontally on the upper chest just under the collar bone, fingers turning inwards towards each other, middle fingertips meeting. Slide your hands away from each other, up and across the shoulders to the back of the neck. Cradle the head in your hands, fingertips meeting.

6. Without stopping, lift your subject's head a few inches from the floor or table and pull from the base of the skull towards you, giving the neck a good stretch. Gently slide your hands up the back of the skull as you allow his or her head to come back down gently. Repeat two or three times (see Fig. 15).

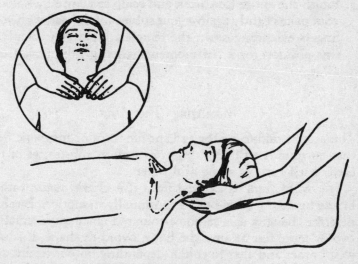

Fig. 15. Stretching the neck.

THE SCALP
Unless your subject is completely bald there is no need to oil the scalp.

1. Lift your subject's head and turn it to the left. Using your fingers, press quite firmly and move fingers *and* scalp over the bone. Try not to simply slide your fingers through the hair over the scalp. Work up and down the head covering the entire area. Repeat on the other side and move the head back to the centre.
2. Run your fingers through your subject's hair several times, allowing your fingers to brush the scalp.
3. Hold your subject's head at the temples, and place your thumbs one on top of the other two or three inches above the hairline. Press quite firmly at 1-inch (2.5cm) intervals back towards the crown as far as you can go.
4. Lightly smooth your hands upwards over your subject's face starting from the chin, over the nose, eyes and forehead and through the hair. Repeat several times.
5. Finish the entire face, neck and scalp sequence by holding your palms lightly against your subject's forehead with your fingers extending down the temples. Hold your hands in this position for a few moments, then gently move them away.

'Massaging' The Aura

The aura is said to be the radiant life-force or magnetic field that surrounds all living things as well as substances of the earth itself such as stone and water.

The word 'aura' is derived from the Greek *avra* meaning breeze because it is said to be continually in motion. Psychics describe the aura as a rainbow-coloured emanation radiating two or more feet around the body, ovoid in shape. It is said to shimmer and alter in colour depending on our health and state of mind. Muddy colours indicate negative emotions or ill health; clear colours are usually a positive sign.

The human aura is composed of three layers: the etheric or vital body which emanates an inch (2.5cm) from the physical body; the astral body, radiating about a foot (30cm) or more around the body; and the mental or spiritual body which can extend to hundreds of yards or metres in certain 'magnetic' people.

The function of the etheric body is to receive and transmit energy or life-force. It is said to leave us in sleep and during meditation. This part of the aura, which is strongest in the hands and feet, can be photographed by a high voltage technique called Kirlian photography. The information captured shows a kind of luminescence and streams of energy flowing from the fingers or toes. To the trained eye, these patterns reflect the emotional and physical state of the individual and can be used as a diagnostic tool.

The astral body, known also as the emotional body, reflects most of the auric colouring. Psychics can often see the auras of women more clearly, probably because they tend to express their emotions more easily than men.

The mental or spiritual body retains all the potential of the individual for his or her future development.

Many of you will choose to dismiss this idea completely out of hand; others may be more open-minded. To the former, I suggest that you read *The Rainment of Light* by David Tansley (Routledge & Kegan Paul 1985), and to the latter that you try out the following experiment.

To see the aura requires a certain amount of clairvoyant ability or esoteric training, but almost all of us can *feel* it to a greater or lesser degree.

Find yourself a willing partner and sit facing each other. Both of you should hold out your hands in front and turn the right palm down and the left palm up. Keep them in this position and place them over the hands of your partner. Close your eyes and become aware of the warmth of your partner's hands. When you feel ready, both of you should raise your right hand above your partner's upturned left hand. Stay there for a few minutes and you will begin to experience one of several sensations: it may be a slight breeze, as the Greek word *avra* indicates, or perhaps a tingling sensation, heat, static or a slight magnetic pull. If you move your right hand slowly back and forth, your partner may experience a curious pulling away sensation or friction as you move your hand towards your body.

To break the contact, move your hands close together again, slide them away and give them a good shake to remove any tingling sensations, or, more precisely, tensions you may have picked up from your partner.

The point of this little exercise is to demonstrate the existence of the healing energy that radiates from the hands of each and every one of us. The more we become aware of its existence, and the more we mediate upon the idea of this energy leaving our hands, the stronger and more useful it will become. Our hands are always more receptive to a person's aura if we have just massaged that person. At the same time, the receiver of massage will also be more receptive to the energy emanating from your hands.

All human beings have the ability to heal, but the person being 'healed' must co-operate by wanting to get better and by 'giving' to the experience. The latter can only be achieved if there is an empathy between giver and receiver.

Before describing auric massage, it is wise to learn how to protect yourself from the emotional and even the physical pains of those you massage. It is not uncommon to feel physically and emotionally drained after giving any kind of massage (physical or auric) to an unhappy person. Therefore, try to carry out the following exercise after every massage.

The most commonly used protective technique practised by healers is the 'White Light' visualization. Follow the instructions for the meditation exercise described in Chapter 1. After you have counted ten breaths as in Step 3, begin to visualize a white light in the sky and imagine it beaming down onto your forehead. Feel it entering your body until you are filled with light. Imagine the light beginning to wrap itself around you until you are cocooned in its radiance. You are inside a white ball of light feeling protected and safe. Once you are safe inside the white light, imagine the beam of light retreating and going back up to the source in the sky.

Water can be used as a protective element. After giving massage of *any* kind, wash your hands under a running tap. If you feel particularly drained or in any way uncomfortable after giving massage, take a shower, if possible, or a bath containing essence of juniper. A drop of juniper essence can also be rubbed into your forearms. Juniper has the power to cleanse psychically as well as physically.

My thanks go to Yves de Maneville, a healer and aromatherapist of many years' experience, for sharing with me his knowledge of juniper.

The aura may be massaged prior to physical massage and/or afterwards. Gently move your hands about 6 inches (15cm) above your partner's body, from the top of the head down to the feet. When you reach the ends of the feet, flick your hands to shake off any physical/emotional tensions. You may concentrate on a particular area of need, such as aching shoulders, if you wish. Your partner may even feel a sensation of warmth or tingling as you pass over his or her body.

Finish the auric massage by gently placing one hand on top of your partner's head and the other at the base of the spine. Stay there until you feel ready to move away.

Self-Massage

When professional treatment or a willing friend are unavailable, you can still derive much benefit from massaging the oils into your own body.

Mix a few teaspoonfuls of massage oil according to your needs or solely because you love its beautiful fragrance. Begin with a bath or shower. The oils will penetrate the skin more readily if it is warm and slightly damp.

The direction of your massage movements should be towards the heart to encourage a good flow of blood, and therefore nutrients, to the area being treated. The only time it is beneficial to massage away from the heart is when you are in a very tense state. It will soothe and calm you to use *very light* stroking movements in a downward direction. Generally speaking, however, you should stroke the skin hand-over-hand in an upward direction. Begin with light strokes and gradually let them become firmer and more vigorous.

Once you have improved the circulation by firm stroking, you may begin gently and rhythmically to knead the fleshy areas of your body, such as thighs and calves. Using each hand alternately, take hold of your flesh with the whole palm of your hand and fingers, pull away from the bones and squeeze as if you were kneading dough. Do not pinch or squeeze so hard that it causes pain; this will do no good at all and may even result in bruising.

When you reach your abdomen, use the whole of your hand and gently and lightly circle the area in a clockwise direction. This helps to prevent constipation by strengthening peristalsis (waves of muscular contraction which move food through the intestines). Incidentally, essential oils are more easily absorbed into the bloodstream when massaged into this area and also the soft skin of the inner side of the thighs and upper arms.

Scalp massage is virtually the same as that described on page 80. If carried out daily for several months, it can help to stimulate hair growth by increasing the circulation and thus nourishment to the hair roots. There is no need to use oil unless you wish to use an aromatherapy oil as a pre-wash conditioning treatment (see 'Hair', Chapter 6).

Shape your hand like a claw and push your fingers firmly into the scalp at the sides. Move in tiny circles, keeping your fingers in the same place so that you move the scalp over the bone rather than simply sliding your fingers across the surface.

Continue all over your head until all parts of the scalp have been reached.

BATHS

The ancients of Egypt, Greece and Rome regarded the ritual of aromatic bathing and anointment with oils as nothing short of a panacea and as necessary to life as food and wine; at least it was for those who could afford such luxury.

One need not be wealthy today to enjoy the luxury and therapeutic value of aromatic baths – unless you delight in fountains of neroli or rose otto!

Essences can be added to your bath simply for pleasure, to aid restful sleep, to help skin disorders, relieve muscular and other pains or to subtly influence your mood. They may be used singly or blended with others.

Sprinkle 3–6 drops of essential oil onto the surface of the water *after* you have drawn your bath; agitate the water to disperse the oil. If you add essential oils as the bath is running, much of the aromatic vapour will have evaporated before you enter the bath. If you have dry skin, you may wish to mix the essences with a few teaspoonfuls of full-fat milk, or in a dessertspoonful of mild liquid soap.
CAUTION: The following essential oils can be highly irritant if you use more than three drops in a bath, especially if you have sensitive skin. These include basil, ginger, fennel, orange and peppermint. These essences should first be mixed in some vegetable oil and the total number of drops made up to 6 with another essential oil. Sandalwood is one of the mildest essences and you may safely use up to 10 drops in your bath. The aroma is very persistent, however, so be sure you really love its sensual, woody aroma!

As a rule of thumb, it is a good idea to use the smallest quantity of essential oil to begin with, increasing the amount if this does not achieve the desired effect.

Children can benefit from aromatic baths too, but please

refer to 'Children and Aromatherapy', page 98. It is vital to use the correct concentrations.

Bath Temperatures

Very hot baths (95-100°F or 35-38°C) can be draining, and if taken frequently will cause the skin to age rapidly. The ideal temperature is around 85-94°F (29-34°C). For a stimulating bath, the water should be cooler (65-70°F or 18-21°C). A bath taken shortly before bed should be tepid (75-85°F or 24-29°C) to help you to sleep.

Footbaths

These can be helpful to ward off chills; for rheumatic or arthritic pain; excessive perspiration, athlete's foot and other skin disorders such as dermatitis. Footbaths are particularly beneficial following reflexology treatment (pressure point massage to the feet) or before ordinary foot massage. The following method for preparing footbaths can also be used as a handbath to treat dry skin conditions.

Sprinkle 3-6 drops of essential oil (diluted in vegetable oil if desired) to a bowl of hand-hot water and steep feet (or hands) for about 15 minutes. Dry them thoroughly and massage into the skin a little oil containing a few drops of the same essence(s).

COMPRESSES

A compress is a valuable way of treating muscular pain, sprains and bruises as well as reducing pain and congestion in internal organs. The compresses can be used hot or cold according to the condition being treated.

For recent injuries such as sprains, bruises, swellings, inflammation and headaches, *cold* compresses are recommended. In the following conditions *hot* compresses are indicated: old injuries, muscular pain, toothache, menstrual cramp, cystitis, boils, abscesses and so forth.

To make a hot compress, sprinkle 4-6 drops of essential oil to about a pint (half a litre) of water as hot as you can bear. Place a small towel or a piece of lint or soft fabric on top of the water. Wring out the excess and place the fabric over the area to be treated. Cover this with a piece of plastic or transparent film then lightly bandage in place if necessary, i.e. for an ankle or knee. Leave in place until it has cooled to body temperature; renew at intervals as required.

For a cold compress, use exactly the same method, but with icy cold water. Leave in place until it warms to body heat and renew as required.

INHALATIONS

These can be used for colds, 'flu, sinusitis, coughs and as a facial steam treatment (see below). The simplest method is to add 2 to 6 drops of essential oil onto a handkerchief and inhale as required. A few drops of the appropriate oil can be sprinkled onto your pillow to ease nasal congestion and to aid restful sleep.

Steam Inhalation

Pour about a pint (half a litre) of near boiling water into a bowl and add two to four drops of essential oil. The quantity depends on the strength of the essence: peppermint, for example, is extremely powerful, whereas sandalwood is very mild. Inhale the vapours for about five minutes, but no longer than ten. To trap the aromatic steam more efficiently drape a towel over your head and the bowl to make a 'tent'.

CAUTION: Steam inhalations should be avoided by asthmatics because concentrated aromatic steam may trigger an attack.

However, warm aromatic baths with a *low* concentration of essential oils (2-3 drops) are recommended.

FACIAL SAUNAS

This method can be used as a facial cleansing treatment. Most skin types benefit from a weekly or fortnightly steaming with the appropriate oils (see page 92). It is particularly good for blemished and congested skins; but must be avoided at all costs if your skin is prone to thread veins. The intense heat will dilate the blood capillaries lying under the skin's surface, thus exacerbating the condition.

Most people use the steaming bowl of water method described previously for facials. However, electric facial saunas are now available. The advantage of these is that only one drop of essential oil is required; more than this will be too overpowering. But a word of warning: American studies on skin health have indicated that over-use (more than once a week over a long period) can cause 'jungle acne', a disorder brought on by the presence of excess moisture in the skin. It seems to me that one should also be wary of too many steamings over a bowl of water too: better to be safe than sorry.

Following the sauna, splash your face with cool water or a skin tonic suitable for your skin type (see Chapter 5).

INTERNAL DOSES

NEVER TAKE ESSENTIAL OILS BY MOUTH: they may damage the stomach lining.

SKIN CARE

A healthy skin is a reflection of good health in general; no amount of external treatment with the finest plant oils will help much if your diet, life-style and emotions are in disharmony. First treat your skin from the inside by following the advice outlined in Chapter 1 (acne and eczema are dealt with separately in Chapter 6).

The chemical structure of essential oils is close to that of the fluids and oils in the skin itself which is why the skin appears to have a natural affinity for them. Essential oils in small quantities diluted in vegetable oil or stirred into a natural plant-based cream (either an unperfumed commercial product or the beeswax recipe in Chapter 5) help to correct skin problems such as premature wrinkling and excessive oiliness or dryness. If the same essences are used in your bath or massaged into your body, enough of the aromatic molecules will be diffused into the bloodstream and lymphatic system to exert a generalised effect from the *inside*. (To understand how the skin absorbs essential oils, see page 33.)

I have discovered that essences used in baths and general massage will help the complexion whether or not they are applied directly to the skin or the face. This is because they work systematically and influence the body as a whole. Very congested or oily skin cannot absorb essential oils efficiently, but when they are used in baths and general massage, they will be more easily absorbed through the softer skin of the abdomen, inner sides of the thighs and upper arms, and, of course, by inhalation of the aromatic vapours.

The basic skin-care regime for all skin-types is as follows:

DAILY
1. Cleansing twice a day. This can be done with a mild pH-balanced soap. Some people prefer to use a cream or lotion cleanser (probably best if you wear make-up). A soapless cleansing bar is the latest innovation and appeals to those who prefer a proper wash with 'soap' and water, but dislike the taut after-feel of soap on their skin. These bars are usually pH-balanced to retain the slight acidic chemistry of the skin's mantle.
2. Apply a skin tonic to freshen the skin, and to remove

residues of soap or cleanser. Oily complexions will benefit from a mild astringent preparation made from rosewater (recipes in Chapter 5).

3. Whilst the skin is still damp, apply a moisturiser made from a natural beeswax and plant oil base (Chapter 5) or a good commercial preparation made from natural plant oils. This will seal in the skin's natural moisture which is constantly escaping into the air. Avoid commercial preparations containing humectants such as glycerin, glycol, sodium pyrrolidone, propylene, or carboxylic acid. Although they make the skin feel good at the time, by attracting moisture from the air, they also tend to attract water from within the outer layers of the skin too. This can easily evaporate, leaving the skin very taut and parchment-like. The skin becomes 'hooked' and will need regular fixes to feel comfortable. As most commercial moisturisers contain these substances, at least half of the female population in western society (and some of its progressive men) must be moisturiser junkies!

WEEKLY

1. To improve the texture of the skin, particularly if you are over thirty, exfoliation is helpful. This will remove the dead cells on the surface of the skin which tend to block the pores causing pigmentation and a dull appearance. Exfoliation will give your skin a lighter translucent appearance. Younger skins tend to shed dead skin cells without help, but as we age the reproductive processes under the skin slow down. New skin cells are formed more slowly and the worn-out cells, which are pushed to the outer layer, tend to stay around in patches.

   Moisten a handful of medium ground oatmeal (ground almonds or cornmeal for very dry skin) and rub into all parts of your face and throat. Be especially attentive around the nostrils. Rinse off with warm to cool water.

2. Facial saunas are discussed on page 88. These are designed to deep-cleanse the skin.

3. A face pack can be applied after a facial sauna or used after ordinary cleansing. They are designed to tone, to stimulate the circulation and to moisturise and/or tighten the skin (recipes for specific skin types will be found in Chapter 5).

Aromatherapy Facial Oils

The most effective way to use essential oils for skin care is to use them as a periodic treatment either once a week or daily for two weeks at a time at monthly intervals. This will prevent your skin from growing accustomed to the essences, and therefore failing to respond positively to them. I am speaking here of direct applications to the face; essences can still be used daily in your bath and as skin perfumes, but remember to alternate your favourite essences at fortnightly or monthly intervals for the best results.

Refer to the following chart for the correct essences for your skin type. Follow the instructions on page 64 for making facial oils, but do not exceed the recommended ½–1 per cent concentrations as too much may irritate your skin. There are various ways of applying the oils for skin treatment.

1. Apply a fine film just after your bath when your skin is still warm and moist. Wipe off any excess after twenty minutes (if necessary) to allow full absorption.
2. Apply half an hour after a face pack or facial sauna.
3. Apply shortly before a walk in the open air (preferably unpolluted country air). The combination of oxygen and essential oils is a superb skin rejuvenator.

If you opt for the once-a-week regime, apply the oils three times a day, otherwise once is enough.

Finally, you can 'doctor' an unperfumed face cream or lotion with the appropriate essence for your skin type. Stir in two or three drops of essential oil to 50g of face cream or one drop to 25ml of lotion and shake well.

ESSENCES TO HELP SPECIFIC SKIN-TYPES

DRY SKIN	OILY SKIN	AGEING SKIN	'NORMAL' SKIN
Camomile	Bergamot	Frankincense	Camomile
Geranium	Cedarwood	Myrrh	Frankincense
Lavender	Cypress	Rose otto	Geranium
Neroli	Eucalyptus	Sandalwood	Lavender
Rose otto	Frankincense		Neroli
Sandalwood	Geranium		Rose otto
Ylang-ylang	Juniper		
	Lavender		
	Lemon		
	Patchouli		
	Rosemary		
	Tea tree		

PUFFY SKIN (excess water)	DEHYDRATED SKIN (parchment-like texture)	ACNE	SENSITIVE SKIN
Cypress	Camomile	Camomile	Try ½ per cent
Geranium	Clary sage	Cedarwood	concentrations
Juniper	Lavender	Cypress	of
Lavender	Rose otto	Eucalyptus	Camomile
Patchouli		Juniper	Lavender
		Lavender	Rose otto
		Patchouli	
		Rosemary	
		Tea tree	

PERFUMES

Many essential oils make delightful skin perfumes when used singly or blended with other essences. They may be used purely for pleasure or to reinforce other aromatherapy treatment – especially when healing distressing states of mind.

Natural perfumes are usually diluted in jojoba oil. In fact, jojoba is actually a liquid wax and, unlike vegetable oil, does not easily go rancid. Commercial perfumes are usually diluted in ethyl alcohol, but this is not generally available (at least in Britain) without a perfumer's licence.

The easiest and perhaps the most economical way to experiment is to put a few drops of your chosen oils on a damp cotton wool stick. If you dislike the aroma, you have only wasted a tiny amount of essential oil. For example, you might like to try one drop of bergamot, one drop of clary sage and two drops of sandalwood. If this aroma is appealing, make into a perfume. Use up to twenty drops of essential oil to a 10 ml base of jojoba. In this instance, you will need five drops of bergamot, five drops of clary sage and ten drops of sandalwood. Store your creations in small dark glass bottles if possible (these are available from many essential oil suppliers).

There need be no rules about blending (though perfumers may disagree) as far as it concerns us in aromatherapy. It is also a matter of personal taste. You may wish to go into technical details about volatility rate, odour intensity, top, middle and base notes, but intuition and a little artistic flair are all that is required. However, with practice, *anyone* can make pleasant blends whether or not they care to acknowledge these two traits.

If you are totally perplexed about blending, remember that 'families' of essences generally harmonize: herbs (basil, clary sage, lavender, marjoram, rosemary), citrus (bergamot, grapefruit, lime), flowers (rose, ylang-ylang, camomile). Other compatible blends are spices with citrus (coriander and ginger with lime) and blends of woody essences (juniper, sandalwood, cedarwood). Woods and resins are a good match too: frankincense with cedarwood is a classic. But why not be wild and creative and mix totally unrelated essences such as frankincense with lavender and lemon; neroli with clary sage; sandalwood with mandarin and ylang-ylang. However, when using very penetrating essences, especially ginger, rose otto and tagetes, go easy – otherwise they will overpower the blend.

Blending is the most creative aspect of aromatherapy and

even a life-time of developing different aromas will not be long enough to experience the myriad of possibilities.

Perfuming Rooms

The most effective way to perfume a room is to use a purpose-designed essential oil burner/vapourizer, or to buy an electric fragrancer. These are now widely available from health shops and essential oil suppliers. A few drops is all you will need for at least an hour of fragrance.

Alternatively, a drop or two on a damp pad of cotton wool or a handkerchief will subtly perfume a room if placed on a radiator. You could also put a drop or two on a *cold* light bulb, so that when you switch on the light, the oil will vapourise into the room with the heat of the bulb. You may prefer to buy a purpose designed fragrance ring, a ceramic or cardboard disc that balances over the top of the light bulb. The essences are dropped on the ring and the warmth from the bulb releases the aromatic vapour.

Room perfuming with essential oils can help to prevent the spread of infection during epidemics. The following essences are the most powerful against air-borne bacteria and make excellent fumigants: pine, thyme, peppermint, lavender, lemon, rosemary, cloves, cinnamon, eucalyptus and tea tree. The last two oils are also credited with anti-viral properties as well, and are useful should a member of the family be stricken with 'flu.

Of course, perfuming rooms with essential oils has a subtle effect on the mood of its occupants. Frankincense, for example, will enhance meditation, yoga practice or a philosophical discussion; orange and cloves will help to jolly-up a winter's party; lavender and neroli will soothe and aid restful sleep at the end of a hectic day. In fact, the possibilities are endless!

AROMATHERAPY DURING PREGNANCY AND CHILDBIRTH

It is important to choose essential oils with care during pregnancy. A few can be toxic, others may induce premature labour if used in high concentrations or taken internally over a period of time. So do not exceed concentrations above 1 per cent (sandalwood is milder and may be used in 2 per cent concentrations if desired). Add no more than four drops of any of the recommended essences to the bath water. To prevent stretch marks, mix a proportion of wheatgerm oil into your massage oil blends (about two teaspoonfuls to five of vegetable oil) or mix 20ml of wheatgerm oil to the basic cream recipe in Chapter 5.

Avoid the following essential oils during pregnancy: basil, cloves, cinnamon, hyssop, juniper, marjoram, myrrh, sage and thyme. Avoid any essence for which you can find little or no information.

The following oils should be avoided during the first trimester of pregnancy because they are too stimulating: fennel, peppermint and rosemary. These oils are acceptable after this period.

Recommended essential oils: bergamot, camomile, coriander, cypress, frankincense, lavender, lemon, mandarin, neroli, patchouli, rose otto, sandalwood, tea tree, ylang-ylang.

After delivery: It may be a good idea to avoid geranium, especially while breastfeeding. This oil may have a stimulating effect on the baby. Also avoid peppermint if breastfeeding as it may decrease the flow of milk. Fennel and lemon grass stimulate the flow of milk.

Massage

Aromatherapy massage is a beautiful way to soothe and reassure both mother and unborn baby. You may carry out all the massage strokes described earlier in this chapter, but with one or two modifications and additions.

1. In late pregnancy, a woman will only be able to lie comfortably on her side for back massage. She may find it more comfortable to bend her uppermost leg and to prop it on a cushion.
2. Start by massaging the lower back using circular strokes with your fingers, then move down and knead her buttocks as well. Pregnant women often hold a great deal of tension in this area.
3. You may like to include *light* clockwise strokes over her abdomen. For this, she should be lying on her back with some cushions or a bolster under her knees to support the lower back. Use slow and caring movements for you are massaging baby as well.

Labour

Essential oils can be an enormous help during childbirth. Lavender massage into the lower back during labour will reduce pain while speeding up the process. During the phase of transition, the shortest yet most painful stage of labour, lavender can be gently and delicately massaged into the abdomen using circular strokes. There should be hardly any pressure attached to this, as it is the lightness of touch that soothes the underlying muscles. Used as a warm compress over the abdomen, lavender will help with the expulsion of the afterbirth.

Some women experience shaking legs at the end of the first stage of labour; if so, massage the thighs by stroking from the upper thigh to the knee and back. Press firmly *down* the leg and lightly as you move your hands upwards. Always keep your movements flowing and rhythmic.

BABIES AND AROMATHERAPY

Your baby will be highly responsive to essential oils and massage because the nervous system and sense of smell in infants is acutely sensitive. Although some aromatherapists advocate the use of essential oils diluted in almond oil for massage, I feel it is safer to use only plain almond, olive, coconut or sesame oil, particularly if your baby is under three months. After this age, you may safely add *one drop* of one of the following essential oils to your baby's bath water; rose, neroli or lavender. Always dilute the essential oil in a few teaspoonfuls of vegetable oil or a dessertspoonful of full-fat milk. Or, better still, use essential oils to perfume the nursery. The simplest method is to add a few drops of essential oil to a damp piece of cotton wool and place it on a radiator. If you have an essential oil burner, scent your baby's room half an hour or so before bedtime. As well as the essences above, you may safely use any of the following for perfuming the nursery, but *do not use on your baby's skin*: bergamot, cypress, lemon, marjoram, frankincense, juniper, orange, camomile.

In recent years, the natural childbirth gurus, headed by such people as Frederick Leboyer and Doctor Michel Odent have revived the ancient art of baby massage. In parts of the East and in many tropical countries, baby massage is regarded as one of the essential skills of motherhood. The technique has been passed down from mother to daughter for centuries. Massage is believed to help babies grow stronger by encouraging deep sleep, better feeding and the relief of colic. Many Western psychologists and paediatricians believe it 'strengthens the bonding and communication between mother and child'. Of course, many enlightened fathers massage their babies too.

CHILDREN AND AROMATHERAPY

Children can enjoy aromatherapy as much as adults, but they are often more discerning in their choice of oils. They tend to choose floral or citrus essences, especially lavender, rose, mandarin and bergamot. However, it is important to use about half the suggested quantities for children under twelve. For example, no more than two or three drops in the bath, and ½ per cent concentrations in massage oils, certainly no more than 1 per cent.

For children under seven, it is advisable to dilute the essential oils in a few teaspoonfuls of vegetable oil or a tablespoonful of full fat milk before adding them to the bath. This will reduce the possibility of neat essential oil being rubbed into the eyes.

Essential oil of lavender is an excellent remedy if added to the bath of a fractious child shortly before bedtime. If the aroma is liked, it will calm and soothe and aid restful sleep. A lavender massage oil applied to the child's back, and over the chest too if he or she is suffering from a cold, will enhance the tranquillizing effect of the bath. When massaging a small child, use quite a light pressure. It is also advisable to avoid using essential oils on the face if your child is under ten. You can, of course, use a little almond or olive oil instead, but keep away from the eye area.

THE ELDERLY

As we grow older, many of us suffer from coldness and stiffness in the joints and the extremities, coupled with poor circulation. Regular massage and aromatic baths will improve skin and muscle tone, flexibility in the joints and the circulation, and may even prevent the onset of hypothermia. CAUTION: You must never massage anyone with cardiovascular disease or if there is inflammation in the joints (as in arthritis). Massage should only be carried out once the inflammation has gone (see 'Arthritis and Rheumatism', 'Circulation', in Chapter 6).

It may be difficult to massage an elderly person on the floor, so unless you have a massage table, you should sit your subject astride on a chair, facing its back. The recipient may lean forward against a cushion if he or she wishes. When you come to work on the lower back, you may have to kneel on the floor or sit in another chair of equal height.

Improving Flexibility and Circulation in Hands and Feet

1. Work in circles with your thumbs over the whole foot or hand, concentrating on the ankle or wrist joint. Work gently and intuitively, always massaging towards the heart.
2. Hold the ankle or wrist with one hand as you *gently* rotate the joint first clockwise then anti-clockwise with the other hand; but *never cause pain*. Regular massage will eventually allow free movement of the joint.
3. Repeat Step 1.
4. To ease stiffness in the finger and toe joints, gently stretch them to their point of resistance, again causing no pain, and rotate first clockwise then anti-clockwise.

When working on the feet, sit close to your subject and support the leg on a cushion placed on your lap, or allow the recipient to rest the foot on a padded stool of a similar height to his or her chair.

The most comfortable way to work on the hands is to sit your subject in an armchair, resting his or her hands on the arms of the chair.

5

Therapeutic Blending and Recipes

The basic methods for using essential oils for general health and skin care are to be found in Chapter 4 where you will also find an essential oil skin-care chart. Before using an essential oil, however, please follow the correct guidelines as outlined here.

1. First try to find the oil, or blend of oils, that best suits your physical and emotional needs. Information about individual oils is to be found in Chapter 3, and in Chapter 6 you will find suggestions for the holistic treatment of a number of common ailments.
2. When choosing an essence to help an emotional state, it is important to be guided by your aroma preference. Although certain oils are believed to be 'stimulating', 'sedative' or 'anti-depressant' (see the chart on page 101), it is not always as straightforward as this. The mind is much more powerful than the aroma of an essential oil. If you dislike the fragrance, no matter what its mood-enhancing properties may be, you are less likely to respond to its charms!
3. MOST IMPORTANT. Before using any essential oil, do check that it is safe for you to use. Certain oils are best avoided during pregnancy, for instance. In Chapter 3 you will find a note headed CAUTION at the end of certain essential oil profiles, should this apply. Most oils should not be used for babies, though a few are safe as room perfumes (see page 97).

PSYCHO-AROMATHERAPY

The following chart categorizes some commonly used essences according to their generally accepted psychotherapeutic effect. However, as mentioned before, this is only a rough guide. Many people respond to the oils in their own unique way.

Those essences described as 'balancing' have the ability to stimulate or relax according to individual needs - a phenomenon totally alien to a synthetic drug. Geranium is perhaps the most remarkable in this respect, but I have known it to be too stimulating for certain sensitive souls.

PSYCHOTHERAPEUTIC CHART

RELAXING	BALANCING	STIMULATING
Camomile	Basil	Black pepper
Clary sage	Citrus oils, especially	Coriander
Cedarwood	bergamot	Eucalyptus
Cypress	Frankincense	Fennel
Juniper	Geranium	Ginger
Lavender	Lavender	
Marjoram	Patchouli	
Myrrh		
Neroli	ANTI-DEPRESSANT	MENTAL STIMULANT
Patchouli		
Rose otto	Basil	Basil
Sandalwood	Bergamot, and other	Coriander
Tagetes	citrus oils	Peppermint
Ylang-ylang	Camomile	Rosemary
	Clary sage	
	Frankincense	
	Geranium	
	Lavender	
	Patchouli	
	Rose	
	Sandalwood	
	Ylang-ylang	

HINTS ON BLENDING

By blending different essential oils, we not only improve the aroma of a single essence, but more interestingly, we can influence the mind-body effect of the oil.

Example 1: You may be feeling depressed and lethargic, yet love the relaxing aroma of sandalwood or cypress. However, you may benefit from a more uplifting fragrance. This could be achieved by blending the sandalwood with a little coriander and bergamot, or the cypress with lavender and geranium, according to your aroma preference.

Example 2: You may be suffering from anxiety and nervous tension as well as aching muscles (as is most common). So you will need a muscle-relaxant, sedative oil such as lavender, marjoram or camomile. To brighten the aroma, try a little ylang-ylang, clary sage, or a touch of rose.

The possibilities are, in fact, endless. There is always a blend to suit the ever changing pattern of mind-body.

RECIPES

BATHS AND MASSAGE OILS
The following blends of essential oils are suitable for therapeutic baths as indicated. To make a corresponding massage oil, simply double the quantity of essential oil and mix with 30ml of a base oil such as almond, sunflower seed or grape seed. Of course, you may wish to adapt the blends to suit your own aroma preference by using more of one essence and less of another. However, try not to exceed the total number of drops suggested.

TO AID RESTFUL SLEEP
Blend 1   Lavender 2, juniper 2, sandalwood 3
Blend 2   camomile 1, neroli 2, clary sage 3
Blend 3   rose otto 1, patchouli 2

FOR MUSCULAR ACHES AND PAINS, COLDS AND FLU
Blend 1   (stimulating) rosemary 3, bergamot 3, ginger 2
Blend 2   (relaxing) lavender 2, marjoram 2, bergamot 2,
           camomile 1
Blend 3   (medicinal aroma) eucalyptus 2, tea tree 3,
           pine 2

FOR TREATING CELLULITE
Blend 1   lemon 3, cypress 2, black pepper 2
Blend 2   cedarwood 4, rose otto 1, patchouli 1
(See also page 125)

Sun Oils

The most effective natural sunscreens are avocado, sweet
almond, sesame, coconut and virgin olive. However, they are
not as protective as the 'high factor' commercial products
available, but are fine for skin that tans easily without burning,
or for an already tanned skin.

RICH
  40 ml sesame oil
  20 ml avocado oil
  10 ml wheatgerm oil
  2 drops of lavender and 2 drops of sandalwood

Funnel the oils into a dark glass bottle and shake well.

LIGHT
  50 ml coconut oil
  20 ml jojoba
  4 drops of lavender *or* 2 drops of camomile

Coconut oil is usually solid at room temperature, so stand the jar in a basin of warm water until it has liquefied, then combine with the other oils. Store in a glass jar.

CAUTION: Never use citrus oils in sun preparations, especially bergamot (unless bergamot F.C.F. – see page 39). These essences may cause skin pigmentation changes when exposed to sunlight.

BASIC CREAM

Home-made skin creams are richer and heavier than the super-light 'mousse' creations available at the cosmetic counter, but they are extremely effective and economical.

This recipe makes a firm set cream which melts on contact with the skin. You will find that a tiny amount will go a long way. Use it as a hand-cream or face-cream for drier skin.

You can experiment with other vegetable oils or blend several as long as they add up to 120ml in all. A portion of wheatgerm oil added to the formula (20ml) will increase its shelf-life and enhance its healing properties.

Store all creams and ointments in a cool dark place and they should keep for at least 2–3 months.

15 g yellow beeswax
120 ml almond oil
45 ml distilled water or rosewater or orange flower water
4–6 drops of essential oil

1. Melt the beeswax with the oil in the top of an enamel double boiler or pyrex basin over a pan of simmering water.
2. Meanwhile, heat the distilled water in another basin over a pan of simmering water.
3. When it has reached the same temperature as the oil (or is hotter), start to add the water, drop by drop at first, to the oil and wax. Beat with a rotary whisk, balloon whisk or an electric food mixer *set at a low speed*.
4. After you have mixed about two teaspoonfuls of the water

into the oil and wax, remove from the heat and continue adding the water a little at a time until you have incorporated it all.

5. As soon as the mixture begins to set, stir in the essential oil.
6. Divide the mixture into little sterilized glass jars and cover tightly.

BASIC OINTMENT (Pomade)

15 g yellow beeswax
60 ml almond oil
10–15 drops of essential oil

Heat the beeswax and almond oil in a double enamel boiler or in a pyrex basin over a simmering pan of water. Stir well, remove from the heat and when it has cooled a little, add the essential oil.

SKIN TONICS

Essential oils are only partially soluble in water, but they can be added to distilled water or flower waters to make very good skin tonics, as long as you remember to shake the bottle before use to disperse the oils.

Skin Tonic Base

300 ml of rosewater, orange flower water or distilled water. For oily skin or acne, you could use a more astringent base such as witch hazel diluted 50/50 with distilled water. Always add 1 or 2 teaspoons of cider vinegar to your blends as this helps to restore the skin's acid/alkali balance, then add 2–4 drops of the appropriate essential oil for your skin type (refer to the skin care chart on page 92). Apply to clean skin once or twice a day.

Aftershave

Commercial preparations often contain alcohol and synthetic fragrance which can irritate sensitive skin. The skin tonic blend suggested above makes an excellent, gently antiseptic, yet pleasantly aromatic aftershave.

Hair Tonics

These are massaged into dry or wet hair once or twice a day. Used regularly, they will improve the condition of your hair and scalp.

For Dandruff

300 ml distilled water or a flower water as suggested for skin tonics, 3 teaspoons of cider vinegar, 6 drops of tea tree, 6 drops of lavender, 3 drops of cedarwood *or* juniper. Pour into a dark glass bottle, and shake well.

For Stimulating Healthy Hair Growth

To the basic flower water or distilled water and cider vinegar base (see previous recipe) add 7 drops of rosemary, 3 drops of sandalwood, 2 drops of patchouli. Pour into a dark glass bottle, and shake well.

MOUTHWASHES

1. For general use:
   300 ml distilled water or 50/50 with witch hazel
   4 drops of lemon
   4 drops of fennel
   4 drops of tea tree

How to use: shake well before use and add two teaspoonfuls of the mixture to a small teacupful of water. Rinse your mouth twice a day after brushing your teeth.

2. For mouth ulcers and other gum disorders:
   30 ml tincture of myrrh
   5 drops of tea tree
   10 drops of cypress
   10 drops of peppermint or fennel

How to use: 6–8 drops in a small teacupful of warm water two or three times a day.

FACE PACKS

For Oily Skin and Acne

1 teaspoon brewer's yeast powder
1 teaspoon natural live yogurt
½ teaspoon warm water (or more if necessary)
1 drop of lavender or juniper or tea tree

Mix the first three ingredients together, then stir in the essential oil. Apply to the face and neck, and leave on for 20 minutes. Rinse off with cool water.

For Dry Skin

¼ of a ripe avocado
1 drop of camomile or rose
About ½ teaspoonful fine oatmeal to bind

Mash the avocado to a pulp and stir in the essential oil. Mix in a little oatmeal to bind. Apply a thin layer to the face and neck, and leave on for 10–15 minutes. Rinse off with tepid water.

For 'Normal' Skin

2 teaspoons natural live yoghurt
1 teaspoon almond oil
1 drop of rosemary or lavender
About ½ teaspoonful of oatmeal to bind

Mix the essential oil into the almond oil and stir into the other ingredients to form a paste. Apply to the face and neck, and leave on for 15-20 minutes. Rinse off with cool water.

6

Remedies for Common Ailments

Aromatherapy can help many disorders, but for the best results it should form part of a holistic health regime. By this I mean that we should look to the prevention of illness, not just to the treatment of symptoms. It is important to remember that illness does not strike 'out of the blue' even though it may seem that way at times. There are many possible causes of ill health; heredity plays a part, but, in the main, its origin lies in our mental state, life-style and diet. So we must seek to cultivate a strong immune system by safe and natural means in order to experience whole health. If the concept of 'holism' is new to you, please read Chapter 1 before referring to the specific remedies outlined in this chapter.

Other forms of gentle therapy such as yoga, medical herbalism and Bach Flower Remedies have been recommended where appropriate, any of which can be used in conjunction with essential oils. Homoeopathy, however, is the exception and is recommended as an alternative therapy should treatment with essences and herbs be only partially effective. Homoeopathic medicine can sometimes be rendered inert or weakened by the powerful aromas of essential oils.

Internal doses of essential oils should be avoided, therefore I have suggested herb teas as an alternative. The basic methods for making these are outlined below. The basic methods for preparing essential oils for external treatment are to be found in Chapter 4 and in the recipe section of Chapter 5.
CAUTION: Where fasting is suggested, do not carry out if you are pregnant, suffer from a heart problem, diabetic, elderly or otherwise very weak. Always seek medical advice first.

PREPARING HERBAL MEDICINES

Infusion: (tea) 14g dried herb to a warmed china or pyrex vessel. Pour over 600ml of boiling water and allow to steep for 10–15 minutes. If you use fresh herb, generally you will need three times as much. Seeds such as fennel or caraway should be bruised before being made into an infusion to release the essential oils from the cells.

Dosage: For general conditions, take a wineglassful three times a day – four-hourly. But do not wake up at night to take any; a good night's sleep is nature's great healer.

Decoction: This is used for hard and woody plant material such as roots, rhizomes and barks. Put 14g of dried plant material, or 42g of fresh, broken into small pieces, into an enamel saucepan or other heatproof vessel. *Never use aluminium* as poisonous seepage will react with the plant alkaloids and its vitamin content, thus damaging the therapeutic properties. Pour over 300ml of water and simmer with the lid on for 10–15 minutes. Strain whilst still hot.

Dosage: Same as infusion.

ACNE

Acne is an infection of the sebaceous glands which shows up as pimples, blackheads and pustules on the face and sometimes on the back, neck, shoulders and chest. Although acne is associated with adolescence, it can occur at any age.

Cause

In teenagers it is almost certainly caused by the hormonal upheavals of puberty, but in adults it may be linked to food allergy. The culprits are very often milk, artificial food additives or wheat. There is also some evidence to suggest that acne may be the result of a disturbance in carbohydrate metabolism and/or inadequate elimination of toxic waste via the alimentary canal.

All types of acne can be exacerbated by a 'junk food' diet high in fat and sugar and lacking in raw, fresh fruits and vegetables. Emotional upset and pre-menstrual syndrome are often implicated.

Treatment

A 60 per cent raw food diet with the addition of the following supplements for about 6 to 12 months: beta-carotene - 30mg (a non-toxic alternative to vitamin A supplements); strong B-complex formula; vitamin C with riboflavonoids - 4×500mg; evening primrose oil (with added vitamin E), especially if PMS exacerbates the condition - 4×500mg; chelated zinc or zinc gluconate - 2×15mg; garlic capsules - four daily. All supplements should be gradually reduced once improvement takes place.

The following herbal teas may be used in combination with the above supplements, or, if finances are limited, you may find them helpful alone with a detoxifying diet. Make up your own herbal blends or drink them separately. Alternate two or three different teas at three-weekly intervals so that your body does not become used to the same one as this can sometimes reduce its effectiveness. Try to get plenty of fresh air and exercise. Moderate sunbathing (up to an hour a day) will also help.

Herb Teas: Dandelion, horsetail *(Equisetum arvense)*, fenugreek, burdock, poke root (decoction), nettle.

All this may appear extremely rigid if you are used to the 'average' western diet of refined foods, low in fibre and high in sugar, salt and fat, washed down with numerous cups of coffee and strong tea. The pressures to conform are great, particularly if you are young; a 'special diet' is often met with ridicule by your peers. You will need much encouragement and emotional support from like-minded parents, friends and relatives. When your skin begins to show marked improvement, some of your more sceptical friends may also decide to embark on a healthier eating regime.

Be sensible, not fanatical. The occasional lapse in your healthy eating plan for social reasons will do no harm provided you return to healthy foods the next day. Worry and anxiety about the food you eat is far more likely to trigger a 'flare up' than the occasional piece of chocolate gateau and cup of coffee.

One word of caution: if your diet is very 'junk food' orientated and almost devoid of the high-fibre wholegrains, seeds, raw vegetables and fruits, do not change your eating habits overnight. Take things slowly, gradually introducing wholefoods into your diet over a period of six months (read the 'Food' section in Chapter 1), otherwise you will experience severe digestive disturbances.

Skin Care: Externally, wash the skin two or three times a day with a soapless cleansing bar or pH-balanced soap, or use a gentle cleansing milk. Afterwards, tone the skin with an appropriate skin tonic (see Chapter 5). If your skin feels taut, apply a fine film of a plant-based, unperfumed moisturiser or a little jojoba with ½–1 per cent concentration of the appropriate essential oil(s) (see below).

Weekly Treatment: If the spots are not oozing, an aromatic facial steam will encourage the release of waste matter. Otherwise, a weekly face-pack will be just as good (see Chapter 5).

Aromatic Baths: Daily or at least three times a week to help eliminate toxins and aid relaxation.

Massage: Back or full body massage once a week if possible, and only if the spots are not oozing. Massage aids the elimination of toxins and promotes deep relaxation.

Other Therapies: Yoga, naturopathy, macrobiotic diet, herbalism, allergy testing. Try homoeopathy if treatment with essential oils has not been helpful after three months.

Essential Oils: Local: tea tree, camomile, camphor, eucalyptus, juniper, lavender, patchouli, rosemary, sandalwood. General (baths, massage, perfumes etc): basil, bergamot, cedarwood, cypress, geranium, lemon, neroli, rose otto.

ANXIETY AND DEPRESSION

Anxiety or depression are perfectly normal responses to harrowing situations; the feelings usually diminish once the crisis is over. Such negative states of mind are only a problem if they become habitual for no apparent reason.

Cause

Anxiety and depression are often the result of stress in its many guises. However, we each respond to stressful situations in our own unique way; what may be a very trying experience for one may simply be a slight irritation to another. Quite often non-specific anxiety or depression can be symptomatic of poor nutrition, food allergy, or simply boredom.

Treatment

First look at your diet and life-style and try to make changes wherever this is feasible (see Chapter 1). Supplement your diet with a strong B-complex formula and about 4×500mg vitamin C, gradually reducing the dosage as you begin to feel better.

Herb Teas: Verbena, camomile, woodruff, lemon balm, lime blossom.

You may also need a reappraisal of your attitudes to life, possibly with the help of psychotherapy, counselling or group therapy.

Aromatherapy reigns supreme as a healing technique to help stress-related disorders. Aromatherapy massage given by a sympathetic and caring person will help enormously by creating ease of mind to enable you to view life more objectively. However, self-treatment with essential oils and other mind/body/psyche techniques such as yoga can be of lasting benefit.

Essential oils are a valuable and safe alternative to the psychotropic drugs and muscle-relaxants used to treat depression and anxiety in orthodox medicine. When using essential oils to subtly alter your emotional state, it is vital to be guided by your perfume preference because we are instinctively drawn to the very oil that most closely corresponds to our present emotional state.

I have attempted to list the most helpful essences, however this is merely a guide; people can vary in their reaction to individual oils or blends of oils. (You may prefer to create your own aroma by mixing two or three oils together.) Use them in baths, massage oils (particularly to the solar plexus area), as vapourizing oils and as skin perfumes.

Other Therapies: Yoga, Tai Chi, meditation, autogenics, Alexander technique, allergy testing, homoeopathy, psychotherapy, counselling, Bach Flower Remedies.

Essential Oils: Citrus oils, camomile, cypress, geranium, lavender, neroli, frankincense, sandalwood, juniper, marjoram, patchouli, rose, clary sage, ylang-ylang, cedarwood, basil, bergamot, coriander.

ARTHRITIS AND RHEUMATISM

There are many forms of rheumatism and arthritis ranging from gout, bursitis and sciatica to rheumatoid arthritis and osteo-arthritis. All forms of the disease are painful and restrict movement to a greater or lesser degree. There may also be inflammation and swelling around the joints as a result of an accumulation of toxins or waste products in the affected tissue.

Cause

Although the causes may be manifold, all natural therapists tend to agree that a diet high in acid-forming and de-natured foods is a major contributing factor in the development of arthritic and rheumatic complaints. Other factors include injury, a cold damp environment and depressive states of mind.

Treatment

This should be a regime of reformed eating habits, sticking to foods of a highly alkaline nature as fár as possible (see below), herbs, essential oils and gentle exercise, preferably yoga. However, if self-treatment offers no relief after about 3-6 months, then it is advisable to seek expert help from a well-qualified natural therapist.

As the ideal diet is a purely personal system of self-healing (no one diet will be right for everyone) it is advisable to take a food allergy test to determine which food substances are particularly harmful to you. Another method is dowsing. Many sufferers use a pendulum to determine whether or not a food is safe for them to eat. Once you are confident with this method, it can be a foolproof system. I recommend the excellent book *Pendulum Power* by Greg Nielson and Joseph Polansky (Destiny Books, 1977; Aquarian Press 1986).

A natural therapist may start you off on a short fast followed by a cleansing diet, but it is advisable to seek professional advice before trying this yourself.

ACID-FORMING FOODS TO BE REDUCED OR AVOIDED
ESPECIALLY IF THEY ARE KNOWN TO EXACERBATE THE
CONDITION
All artificially-preserved 'foods' in packets and cans. Refined carbohydrates – white bread, sugar etc. Red meat and pork products. Red wine. Rhubarb. Gooseberries. Black and redcurrants. Spinach. Vinegar (but not always cider vinegar). Dairy products. Eggs. Spices. Coffee. Black tea. Alcohol, particularly red wine, port and sherry.

It is advisable to cut down on salt, as this contributes to the accumulation of toxins.

ALKALINE-FORMING FOODS GENERALLY REGARDED AS
GOOD, ALTHOUGH YOU MAY FIND THAT SOME OF THESE
CAUSE PROBLEMS TOO

Apples	Tomatoes	Bean and seed sprouts
Raspberries	Peaches	(particularly alfalfa)
Grapefruit*	Nectarines	Green beans
Lemons*	Cherries	Watercress
Oranges*	Strawberries	Celery
Raisins and all dried fruit	Apricots	Green peas
Papaws	Bananas	Lettuce
Pineapple	Green grapes	Carrots

* Although these are 'acid' fruits, they become alkaline during digestion.

EAT IN MODERATION
   Fish   Pulses
   White meat   Nuts
   Wholegrain products   Seeds

Dietary Supplements: Many people have found that the green-lipped mussel extract (available in tablet form) is very helpful in reducing inflammation, but it should be used in conjunction with dietary reform as the relief from pain may eventually turn out to be short-lived. However, green-lipped mussel extract should be avoided by those suffering from an allergy to shellfish. Another beneficial supplement is kelp. All sufferers should take at least 500mg of vitamin C a day, unless it causes diarrhoea.

Baths: To speed the elimination of toxins from the system via the skin (mainly uric acid), fairly hot Epsom salts baths (95°F or 35°C) should be taken once a day for a week and then on alternate days until there is a marked improvement; thereafter, take an Epsom salts bath once a week. Dissolve 450g (1 lb) of Epsom salts in a few pints of boiling water and add to your bath. Relax for about 10–15 minutes, but do not use soap as this interferes with the beneficial action of the salts.

Caution: Not to be taken by anyone with high blood pressure or a heart condition. Elderly or very frail people should use 225g (½ lb) of Epsom salts to start with, gradually increasing as the bath becomes better tolerated.

You may add appropriate essential oils to the water if you wish, but this may be merely for aesthetic purposes as the skin cannot absorb the essences if it is busy throwing off toxic wastes. I personally feel they are more beneficial rubbed into the skin an hour or two after the bath. By all means use essential oils in your bath for therapeutic purposes between the Epsom Salts baths. It is extremely important to move the joints as much as possible after massage or hot baths to prevent congestion which will make matters worse.

Massage: This is helpful if there is no inflammation; if you are unsure, seek medical advice. The most effective way to reduce inflammation and swelling is to alternate hot and cold essential oil impregnated compresses. Always end with a cold compress to prevent the hot application from having an enervating effect upon the skin (see Chapter 4 for instructions on making compresses).

Herb Teas: Yarrow, meadowsweet, celery seed (decoction), devil's claw (decoction or in tablet form), black cohosh, honeysuckle flowers, dandelion, burdock, nettle.

Other Therapies: Sunshine, swimming, fresh air and salt water are a wonderful healing combination, so whenever you can, enjoy them to the full. Yoga, osteopathy, chiropractic, Alexander technique, medical herbalism, acupuncture, food allergy testing, naturopathy, homoeopathy.

Essential Oils: Camomile, camphor, eucalyptus, lemon, rosemary, juniper, cypress, coriander, marjoram, lavender, ginger.

ATHLETE'S FOOT

This is a fungal infection between the toes, associated with warm, moist conditions. It may also appear on other parts of the body in the form of an itchy rash known as ringworm.

Cause

Excessive perspiration in poorly ventilated footwear invites infection which can also be picked up in the changing rooms of public swimming pools or sports centres.

Treatment

Allow your feet to breathe by exposing them to sunshine and fresh air whenever possible. Keep them scrupulously clean and dry. Apply a few drops of neat lavender or tea tree essence to the sore parts. Severe cases, involving the toenails and other areas of the foot (fissured heels is a symptom), need to be treated holistically. A course of B-complex and dietary reform may need to be implemented. Also, footbaths (twice daily if possible) containing 5-6 drops of an appropriate essential oil and a tablespoon of cider vinegar (instructions for preparing footbaths are to be found in Chapter 4). Then apply an essential oil ointment: to 30 gm of an unperfumed commercial preparation, add 15 drops of tea tree, lavender or a blend of essences.

Essential Oils: Patchouli, lavender, lemon, tagetes, peppermint, tea tree.

BOILS

Boils are indicative of a run-down condition as a result of physical neglect or emotional disharmony.

Treatment

Changes in life-style and diet (see Chapter 1). To rid the body effectively of boils, seek to stimulate the body's defences by internal and external treatment with herbs and essential oils. You may also need an extra boost from the following supplements: vitamin B-complex, 4×500mg vitamin C, 4 garlic capsules a day, gradually reducing the dosages as the condition improves.

Herb Teas: Burdock, yellow dock, poke root (decoction), pasque flower.

Compress: To draw out pus from the boil, apply a hot compress of camomile essence, followed by an ointment or cream containing the appropriate essence(s).

Essential Oils: Camomile, lemon, lavender, myrrh, tea tree.

BREASTFEEDING PROBLEMS

Many mothers worry endlessly and often unnecessarily about the quantity and quality of their milk. If you are a breastfeeding mother and have a good wholefood diet, are free of major stress, chronic illness and your life-style allows for adequate rest, fresh air and exercise, then you should experience few problems.

If your baby is constantly fretful or listless and fails to gain a reasonable amount of weight, there may be genuine cause for concern, so you must seek professional advice. Breastfed babies, however, tend to grow more slowly and often weigh less than bottle-fed babies. This is because cows' milk contains nearly three times as much protein as that found in human milk. A baby needs much less protein than a calf because the growth rate of the human infant is very slow compared to other animals. Calves are running around soon after birth, whereas babies take one or two years to develop sufficient strength in their legs to walk. This may explain the accelerated growth rate of many bottle-fed babies.

Breast milk, particularly the early milk of the first few days called colostrum, contains high amounts of vitamins and antibodies which help to protect the baby against many viral and bactericidal diseases. Breastfeeding also offers a higher protection against allergic disorders such as eczema and asthma. But I do not wish to sow seeds of doubt and guilt in those few women who genuinely cannot breastfeed for one reason or another. Many bottle-fed babies thrive beautifully, especially if they are eventually weaned onto a well-balanced wholefood diet and are given plenty of love.

Herbs to Stimulate Milk Flow: Fennel, caraway, dill, fenugreek, goat's rue, milk thistle.

Essential Oils: Baths and massage; fennel (no more than three drops), lemon grass.

Note: The herb tea and the essential oil of peppermint and sage *decrease* milk flow.

Sore or Cracked Nipples

One of the finest essences for healing sore or cracked nipples is rose otto. It is best applied in a beeswax cream or ointment as described in Chapter 5. Use up to eight drops in the recipes and apply at least three times a day, but wash the nipples before feeds and reapply afterwards.

A very amusing, yet ingeniously successful way to allow sore nipples to heal without depriving the baby of breast milk was recommended to a friend of mine by the local midwife: cover the nipple with a rubber teat from a baby's bottle during feeds. The baby will draw milk from the breast through the teat without causing the mother any discomfort at all!

Essential Oils: Rose otto, camomile.

BRONCHITIS

Bronchitis is an infection of the bronchial tubes that lead to the lungs. Symptoms are a chesty cough (the body's attempt to expel the mucus), a high temperature, chest pains and irritation between the shoulder blades.

Cause

Tobacco smoke, a mucus-forming diet, inadequate breathing, air pollution, poor posture, stress and sometimes allergy (especially if you are prone to bronchitis). The digestive and circulatory systems and also the kidneys and skin may be functioning poorly, thus there is a heavier burden on the lungs to eliminate waste. The condition is exacerbated by cold damp air.

Treatment

The best approach is to fast on fruit juice diluted 50/50 with spring water, herb teas and plain spring water for about 24 hours (under medical supervision). If your digestive system can take it, this should be followed by a day or two on just fruit, mainly apples, grapes and citrus fruits; avoid dried fruits and bananas. During the fast and semi-fast, take a daily aromatic bath with the appropriate essential oils and make a massage oil to rub into your chest and back. Gradually wean yourself onto a largely raw food diet as free as possible from dairy products and starchy foods as these are highly mucus-forming (see also the section on food in Chapter 1). You should also look to your life-style and make some necessary changes wherever this is feasible.

Steam inhalations using oils such as eucalyptus and sandalwood should be carried twice a day for a few days until there is marked improvement. Burn essential oils in your bedroom or use a room-spray to help purify the air.

Supplements: Take the following supplements daily, particularly during the winter months: 4×500mg vitamin C, strong B-complex formula, 2-4 garlic capsules. Gradually reduce as improvement takes place.

Herb Teas: Thyme, eucalyptus, coltsfoot, lungwort, hyssop, white horehound.

Other Therapies: Yoga, Alexander technique, osteopathy, chiropractic, naturopathy, medical herbalism, food allergy testing, deep breathing exercises.

Essential Oils: Garlic (capsules), camphor, eucalyptus, lavender, peppermint, rosemary, sandalwood, cedarwood.

BRUISES

Apply a *cold* compress, an ointment or an oil containing the appropriate essence(s). Comfrey or arnica ointments are also excellent for bruises.

Essential Oils: Camphor, ginger, fennel, tea tree.

BURNS AND SCALDS

Cool the skin under cold running water as soon as possible. Apply a few drops of *neat* lavender oil to small burns or make a cold compress for larger burns (see Chapter 4). To prevent scarring, apply an oil, cream or ointment (Chapter 5) containing at least 15 per cent wheatgerm oil and the correct number of drops of lavender essence. Keep this up for about a month for the best results.
SERIOUS BURNS SHOULD BE REPORTED TO YOUR DOCTOR IMMEDIATELY.

Sunburn

Take a cool bath with about four tablespoonfuls of cider vinegar and up to ten drops of essential oil; lavender is a good choice. Afterwards, apply an oil, cream or ointment (Chapter 5) containing wheatgerm oil or any of the essences listed below. For very sore patches, it is less painful to paint on the massage oil with a small, soft-bristle brush.

Essential Oils: Camomile, eucalyptus, geranium, lavender, rosemary, tea tree.

CATARRH

Naturopaths have always maintained that catarrh is a result of a build-up of toxic matter that the body is forced to eliminate.

Cause

Faulty nutrition, stress and sometimes allergy.

Treatment

Look to your diet and life-style and take steps to reduce the amount of stress in your day to day living (Chapter 1). Cut out the most mucus-forming foods for at least six months; these include dairy products and refined carbohydrates such as white bread, flour and sugar. 'Junk foods', of course, should be avoided like the plague for they place an enormous burden on the liver and kidneys to eliminate their many additives.

To initiate the healing process, a fast should be undertaken but only under the guidance of a qualified therapist. The general diet should consist of at least 60 per cent raw salads, fruits and seeds. For three to six months you may need the following supplements to combat the stress placed on the body during the detoxification period: B-complex, 4×500mg vitamin C and a multi-mineral supplement. Taper off gradually as improvement takes place.

Take four garlic capsules daily. All the following can be carried out at home: steam inhalations, drops on a handkerchief to inhale as desired, baths and massage oils to be rubbed into the chest at night. Regular aromatherapy massage will help to eliminate toxins and promote deep relaxation.

Take any of the following herb teas three times a day: peppermint, camomile, elderflower, yarrow, lemon balm or ginger (decoction).

Other Therapies: Yoga, allergy testing, herbalism, naturopathy, homoeopathy.

Essential Oils: Lavender, peppermint, rosemary, myrrh, camomile, frankincense, marjoram, sandalwood, eucalyptus, cedarwood.

CELLULITE

This is an accumulation of dimpled, stubborn fat which occurs mainly on the thighs, buttocks, hips and upper arms. If the area is pinched, the skin puckers and ripples and does not immediately spring back into place. The affected areas have an orange peel appearance and are cold to the touch. Unlike ordinary fat tissue, cellulite contains a large proportion of water and tissue wastes.

Cause

Many cases are almost certainly hormone-linked. Some women produce large quantities of oestrogen which is not balanced out by optimum levels of its antagonist hormone progesterone. According to Doctor Pierre Dukan in his book *La Cellulite en Question* (La Table Ronde, Paris 1983), 75 per cent of cellulite sufferers found the condition started during periods of hormonal upheaval such as pregnancy, the menopause, puberty and when first taking oral contraceptives.

A misaligned spine can create muscle spasm and pressures on nerves and blood vessels in the lower back. If left unchecked, these pressures can contribute to cellulite by hindering lymphatic drainage. Alexander technique, osteopathy or chiropractic can be used in conjunction with aromatherapy and diet to realign the spine and eliminate the pressures in the spinal area.

Other known causes include stress, an additive-laden diet,

constipation, poor circulation, a sedentary life-style, faulty liver, kidney, lung or digestive functioniong.

Treatment

First and foremost look carefully at your diet and try to eliminate the worst offenders. These include all refined and processed foods laden with chemical additives, sugar and white flour products; salty foods such as smoked fish and preserved meat products; coffee, alcohol, and to a slightly lesser degree tea.

A largely raw, wholefood diet is to be recommended (see Chapter 1). Drink copious amounts of natural spring water to flush out the kidneys. You may need to undergo a two or three day fast or semi-fast to start off the detoxification programme, but this is best carried out under the supervision of a qualified natural therapist with a sound knowledge of dietetics.

Herb Teas: The following herbs are particularly good for cellulite sufferers because they are natural diuretics and are renowned by herbalists as 'blood purifiers': nettle, golden rod, dandelion, meadowsweet.

Fresh air and exercise, correct breathing and daily relaxation are as important as good nutrition (see Chapter 1).

Regular stimulating massage with the appropriate essential oils will help to break down toxic deposits, improve circulation and encourage adequate lymph drainage. Although professional aromatherapy/lymphatic massage is extremely effective, self-treatment such as frictioning with a loofah and massaging the affected areas with suitable essences can be helpful (follow the self-massage technique described in Chapter 4).

Other Therapies: Yoga, Tai Chi, naturopathy and hydrotherapy, Alexander technique, osteopathy, chiropractic.

Essential Oils: Cypress, lemon, juniper, rosemary, lavender, geranium, fennel, patchouli, cedarwood.

CHILBLAINS

Chilblains are an inflammatory condition of the skin, whereby the affected part becomes swollen and itchy, sometimes leading to ulceration. Chilblains generally occur on the toes and fingers, sometimes the ears and nose.

Cause

Exposure to cold winds, coupled with poor circulation and sometimes calcium and silicon deficiency.

Treatment

As a preventative measure, use regular massage of the hands and feet and pinching of the outer edges of the ears to stimulate the circulation. The following herb teas are helpful as a preventative measure as well as treatment from the inside: nettle - rich in minerals, horsetail (*Equisetum arvense*) - rich in silicon, anti-inflammatory.

Ointment: Follow the basic recipe for an ointment or a cream as in Chapter 5, and add 6 drops of any one of the essential oils listed below.

Broken Chilblains: Foot or hand baths with lavender essence. Pierce a garlic capsule and paint the contents onto the affected parts (if you can stand the smell!).

Essential Oils: Lavender, lemon, camphor.

CHILDHOOD ILLNESSES

Nowadays, these are generally quite controllable and not at all serious if diet, hygiene and social conditions are adequate. It does appear to be a fact of life that the young are susceptible to all manner of germs and viruses. This is nature's way of strengthening the immune system. Complications are only likely to arise if the child has a congested immune system. This is avoided by a good wholefood diet (as outlined in Chapter 1), fresh air, exercise, adequate housing and, above all, love. Sadly, many children in the world today are deprived of these basic requirements, so lasting health and happiness are bound to be in jeopardy.

Treatment for all illnesses is largely dietary with external applications of essential oils and sometimes room sprays to prevent the spread of infection.

If a child's appetite has diminished, all well and good; a 24-hour fast is the most appropriate treatment. During a fast, plenty of fresh water should be taken as required until the appetite begins to return. A day or so on a diet of fresh fruit and fruit juice (preferably grape) diluted 50/50 with spring water should precede a gradual return to a wholefood diet.

Children can benefit from skilful use of essential oils in a myriad of common ailments. Anything from coughs and colds to earache and measles can be soothed with an aromatic remedy. Essences can be used in baths, inhalations, compresses, massage oils, creams or ointments in concentrations of about half that recommended for adults in Chapter 4. However, I must admit that I usually refer parents to a qualified homoeopath if a child is under the age of five years, or if the ailment is of a chronic nature.

Chickenpox

In children the disease is a mild fever which begins with the appearance of blisters on the chest and back. These later spread to the rest of the body and cause severe itching.

Treatment

Follow the dietary advice as for measles, unless your child is only mildly affected and has a ravenous appetite! Add any of the recommended essences to his or her bath using half the usual number of drops. For children under six, it may be safer to mix the essences into a little vegetable oil. If the scalp is affected as well, add about 6 drops of essential oil to a large basin of warm water and pour over your child's hair, taking great care to avoid the eyes. Repeat the bath and hair rinse twice a day until the spots begin to diminish. To relieve itching between the baths, make up the following lotion and sponge the skin as required: 100 ml distilled water, 50 ml witch hazel, 3 drops camomile, 3 drops lavender, 4 drops eucalyptus. Shake well and dilute 50/50 with warm water before use.

Other Therapies: Medical herbalism, homoeopathy.

Essential Oils: Camomile, lavender, eucalyptus.

German Measles

German measles - or *rubella* - is a much milder version of measles. Your child will manifest symptoms of a feverish cold, mild aches and pains and tender lymph nodes in the neck. The rash appears on the first or second day, and lasts for about three days.

If you are a pregnant woman and have not had *rubella* but have been exposed to the disease, it is vital that you consult a homoeopathic doctor as soon as possible. *Rubella* can be dangerous to unborn babies. You may be given a homoeopathic dose of *rubella* itself (called a nosode) or gamma globulin injections may be indicated.

Treatment: As for measles.

Measles

Your child may first lose his or her appetite and complain of a headache. Soon a feverish cold develops accompanied by a sore throat and a dry cough. The eyes will be red and sensitive to light. Over the next few days a red rash appears spreading downwards over the body. The illness usually lasts a week, but complications can occur in babies, so it is advisable to seek medical advice, preferably from a homoeopathic doctor.

Treatment

Put your child to bed in a dimly-lit, but well-ventilated room. Allow plenty of spring water to drink, but nothing else (except fruit if hungry) for about twelve to twenty-four hours. This should be followed by a day or two on an all fruit diet with the addition of any of the following fruit juices diluted 50/50 with spring water: grape, lemon (sweetened with honey or fructose), orange. However, do seek medical advice as well.

Herb Teas: Peppermint (but not if taking homoeopathic medicine as it will antidote the effect), elderflower, lemon balm.

Older children may be able to swallow a garlic capsule once a day during the recovery period or once the fever has subsided. Otherwise a bowl of garlic soup for lunch or supper for a week or more will be as effective.

Eucalyptus is regarded as a specific for measles and should be used in the bath, as a lotion and as a fumigant: *Lotion* – 50 ml witch hazel, 50 ml distilled water, 10 drops of eucalyptus. Sponge the body frequently with this lotion. *Fumigant* – 150 ml water, 10 drops of eucalyptus, 10 drops of thyme, 5 drops lavender. Put into a house plant spray or atomiser and fumigate the room two or three times a day or vapourize the oils in an essential burner.

Other Therapies: Medical herbalism, homoeopathy.

Essential Oils: Eucalyptus, camomile.

Mumps

This is normally a mild childhood illness, but it can be severe in adults and older children. Symptoms are painful swelling of the salivary glands on one or both sides of the face. In males, the testicles may also become swollen and, in some cases, this can lead to sterility.

Treatment

Bed rest and a fluid diet of fruit or vegetable juices and spring water if chewing is painful.

In older children, the following mouthwash is helpful to combat the infection if used two or three times a day: 100 ml distilled water, 10 drops of lemon essence, 3 drops of camomile essence. Shake the bottle well before use and add two or three teaspoons of the mixture to a teacup of warm water. Do not swallow the mouthwash.

Apply gently to the affected areas a massage oil containing either of the recommended essences in a ½ per cent dilution.

Other Therapies: Homoeopathy, medical herbalism.

Essential Oils: Camomile, lemon.

CIRCULATION (POOR)

Good circulation depends upon adequate exercise, correct breathing and good nutrition (see Chapter 1).

Treatment

As well as the above, aromatherapy massage is one of the finest preventative therapies for poor circulation and its associated problems such as cramp, chilblains, and, more seriously, varicose veins and even hypothermia in the elderly and the very young. During massage, blood and lymph pass much more rapidly through the body. The pulse rate drops as the heart slows. Although the local blood flow is increased, the burden on the heart is decreased; blood pressure is lowered and overall relaxation of body and mind is experienced as a result.

Herb Teas: Thyme, yarrow.

Other Therapies: Yoga, reflexology, medical herbalism.

Essential Oils: In massage and as drops in your bath: black pepper, juniper, cypress, marjoram, lavender, rosemary, coriander, camphor, orange.

COLDS

A cold is an upper respiratory viral infection affecting the nasal passages and throat.

Cause

Although we are said to 'catch a cold' from other sufferers or as a consequence of drastic temperature changes it is more accurate to say that we have created a crisis in our body toxicity level as a result of poor nutrition and/or emotional disharmony. Stress of any kind appears to weaken the immune system leaving us vulnerable to cold viruses no matter how sound our diet may be.

Treatment

Conventional medicine offers no cure for the common cold, but Doctor Linus Pauling, the Nobel Prizewinner, has discovered that megadoses of vitamin C, if taken early enough at the onset of the cold symptoms, will, in fact, stop the virus in its tracks. The dose is very large indeed; 500 mg every two hours for twelve hours. Vitamin C is rather like a contraceptive for cold viruses. When the body is saturated with this vitamin, the virus only goes through one cycle of growth instead of several. This remedy does not suit everyone, however; it may cause diarrhoea or even a skin rash. For these people and for those who have left it too late, aromatherapy and herbal preparations will do much to relieve the symptoms.

A short fast is the naturopathic approach to infections, but do seek medical advice first. A fruit and salad diet along with copious amounts of hot herbal teas and lemon and honey drinks is the next best thing.

Herb Teas: Camomile, coltsfoot, elderflower, peppermint, yarrow.

Steam inhalations, aromatic baths, drops on a handkerchief and on your pillow will help to clear the respiratory passages and will prevent the infection travelling to the sinuses.

If you have young children at home, it is a good idea to spray the house two or three times a day with essential oils, or use an essential oil burner. For a plant-spray bottle, put the following mixture into 150 ml of water: ten drops of eucalyptus, five drops of lemon, five drops of pine, cloves or tea tree. Shake well before use.

During the winter months, take two or three garlic capsules a day as a safeguard against infections. Ensure that you are getting enough vitamin C and B-complex. If you live or work in a polluted environment, you may need to supplement your diet with 500 mg of vitamin C and a strong B-complex formula to boost your immune system.

Essential Oils: Black pepper, ginger, cinnamon bark (as a fumigant only, this oil must never be used on the skin), cedarwood, eucalyptus, tea tree, basil, camphor, melissa, lavender, lemon, pine, orange, peppermint.

CONJUNCTIVITIS

Conjunctivitis is an inflammation of the eyelid, caused by a poor diet deficient in vitamins A, C and B-complex.

Treatment

Increase all foods rich in the above nutrients; these include carrots, oily fish, fresh fruits and seed sprouts, whole grains and brewer's yeast. You may even need to take a multi-vitamin and mineral supplement for a while, especially if you are prone to conjunctivitis.

In my opinion, essential oils should *never* be applied to the eyes, no matter how diluted; they may burn the delicate eye tissue. It is far safer and very effective to apply rosewater or a lotion made from a herb tea (and allowed to cool) such as camomile, eyebright or elderflower. If you can find a herbal supplier selling tinctures of the above plants, these are much easier to use. Put six drops into 120 ml of luke-warm water and apply as a compress (cotton wool pads) or in an eye bath.

CONSTIPATION

Naturopaths have always extolled the virtues of a wholefood diet as a preventative of constipation and many other 'diseases of civilization' such as appendicitis, diverticulitis and even bowel cancer.

In recent years, this seemingly simple approach has finally gained some credence in the orthodox profession. Many eminent doctors and nutritionists, notably Dr Denis Burkett, have published their findings on the importance of fibre in the diet to promote normal functioning of the digestive tract.

Although constipation is largely the result of a fibreless diet, a sedentary life-style and emotional disharmony are often the root cause. Steps should be taken to reduce and manage the inevitable stresses of life by making certain life-style alterations where this is feasible (see Chapter 1).

The elderly and the disabled are often forced to lead a sedentary life, and as a result are usually prone to constipation. Daily abdominal massage with essential oils, using gentle clockwise strokes, should be carried out in conjunction with a wholefood diet, deep breathing (preferably in the fresh air) and, if possible, gentle physiotherapy or body massage.

Drink plenty of pure water – at least six glasses a day. One or two glasses of warm water before breakfast will flush out toxins.

Herb Teas: Camomile, centuary, dandelion, strawberry.

Other Therapies: Yoga, naturopathy, medical herbalism, homoeopathy.

Essential Oils: To be used in baths and massage: fennel, marjoram, rosemary, black pepper, rose.

COUGHS

A cough is the body's attempt to clear the air passages of irritating mucus, bacteria, dust, pollen or smoke.

Cause

Coughs often accompany other infections, such as colds and

'flu, so follow the treatments outlined for the specific ailment. Whooping cough is a serious illness and should be treated by a well-qualified medical herbalist, homoeopath, or orthodox doctor (preferably a person with a holistic approach).

Treatment

Drink plenty of spring water, fruit juices (diluted 50/50 with spring water) and any of the herb teas recommended below. Dairy products and refined starches should be cut down to a minimum, particularly if you have a thick mucousy cough. Garlic, eaten raw in salads or taken as soup can be helpful, but it is important to realise that *garlic may be contra-indicated if you have a dry cough* (seek the advice of a qualified natural therapist if you are unsure).

Herb Teas: Coltsfoot, marshmallow, mullein, honeysuckle flowers, elecampane. For dry coughs, the best remedies are coltsfoot and wild lettuce.

Two drops of any of the essences listed below can be mixed in a teacupful of water and used as a gargle three times a day. Any of the recommended oils may be rubbed into the throat and chest at night (in a 2–3 per cent concentration mixed with vegetable oil, or 1 per cent for children over five years). Babies and very young children are best treated homoeopathically.

Persistent coughs lasting more than two weeks, despite treatment with herbs, diet and essential oils, should always be investigated by a qualified natural therapist or a doctor.

Other Therapies: Medical herbalism, naturopathy, homoeopathy.

Essential Oils: Cypress, eucalyptus, juniper, peppermint, sandalwood, lavender, tea tree, cedarwood.

CYSTITIS

Cystitis is an inflammation of the bladder due to infection. If not treated properly it can damage the kidneys. The symptoms are burning pains when passing urine and a frequent desire to do so. If there is blood or pus in the urine, medical help should be sought immediately.

Cause

Many conditions predispose towards cystitis and only a medical examination and laboratory urine tests can ascertain the cause. Although cystitis mostly occurs in women, men are by no means immune. Those who have undergone surgery involving the urethra or who suffer from an enlarged prostate gland are more likely to suffer attacks of cystitis. The enlarged gland may press on the bladder causing a little urine to be trapped in a 'back pocket' where it soon becomes a breeding ground for bacteria.

In women, pressure from a back-tilting uterus may also result in incomplete emptying. An osteopath is the best person to consult if this condition is suspected or has been confirmed by medical examination. However, treatment with essential oils and the dietary regime outlined below should be carried out as well.

Cystitis may also be triggered by stress and sometimes industrial chemicals or paint fumes.

So-called 'honeymoon cystitis' may occur after a bout of prolonged sexual activity. The best preventative remedy is to drink a glass of water immediately after sex and to empty the bladder as soon as possible.

Treatment

Flush out the kidneys with copious amounts of camomile tea, apple juice diluted 50/50 with spring water or just plain warm water. Your diet should lean heavily on the alkaline-forming foods such as fruits and vegetables. Take lashings of live yoghurt; about 700 ml a day. If you really cannot face that amount or have an allergy to dairy products, then try acidophilus tablets (yoghurt bacteria) if you can find them. However, some of these preparations can be very expensive.

Aromatherapy treatment consists of warm compresses over the lower back, massage and aromatic baths.

Other Therapies: Chiropractic, osteopathy, yoga, Alexander technique, medical herbalism, naturopathy, homoeopathy.

Essential Oils: Bergamot, camomile, cedarwood, eucalyptus, juniper, lavender, pine, sandalwood.

EARACHE

Earache often accompanies a cold or 'flu brought on by the spread of infection from the throat to the eustachian tube in the ear. Occasionally, an earache may be a symptom of middle-ear infection, so persistent earache must be investigated by a doctor, homoeopath, or perhaps a medical herbalist without further delay.

Treatment

Warm an eggcupful of olive or almond oil and add *one* drop of any of the essences listed below. Using a medicine dropper, put a few drops into the ear and seal it in with a small ball of cotton wool.

Essential Oils: Camomile, rosemary, lavender, peppermint.

ECZEMA

This is an itchy, scaly and fissured inflammation of the skin sometimes characterised by a sticky fluid discharge.

Cause

Many sufferers have a family history of eczema or other allergy-related disorders such as asthma and hayfever. Allergy to certain food substances as well as household and industrial chemicals is almost certainly implicated. However, the major part of the problem is within the personality of the sufferer – the condition flaring up during periods of stress.

Treatment

It is advisable for all sufferers to have an allergy test. Not everyone will be allergic to the same substances, but all sufferers should avoid dairy products as far as possible. The importance of a wholefood diet consisting of plenty of raw salads, fruits and sprouted grains/seeds/legumes cannot be over-emphasised.

Many people have benefited from a course of evening primrose oil (Efamol). The average dose may vary according to individual needs, but is about 4×500 mg a day. You may also need a good B-complex formula and 2×500 mg of vitamin C as well.

The following herb teas are recommended: camomile, red clover, nettles, chickweed, marigold.

Essential oils may be used in baths, massage oils and in home-made creams and ointments (Chapter 5). Start with camomile alone for dry eczema, or a blend of camomile/juniper for weeping eczema. It is always best to start off with the lowest concentration of essential oils – ½ per cent.

Regular aromatherapy massage will have far-reaching effects by releasing much deep-rooted tension, thus allowing the body to respond more readily to natural treatments.

Other Therapies: Allergy testing, herbalism, naturopathy, homoeopathy, yoga, meditation, Bach Flower Remedies.

Essential Oils: Camomile, lavender. Weeping eczema: Juniper.

GUMS

Dentists are always telling us that more teeth are lost as a result of gum disease rather than dental decay. If we look after our gums, our teeth will look after themselves.

Gingivitis

The gums bleed when they are brushed or when hard or fibrous foods are eaten. This is largely the result of an invisible bacteria called plaque which hardens as a result of enzymes in saliva and forms a hard calculus deposit known as tartar. Tartar can eventually force the gum away from the bony socket; food particles become lodged in the crevices and are attacked by bacteria. If left unchecked, this can lead to severe gum disease – pyrrhoea.

Treatment

A well-balanced wholefood diet, scrupulous dental hygiene and the use of dental floss. Visit your dentist every six months for a check-up. Use the tincture of myrrh mouthwash described in Chapter 5.

Mouth Ulcers

An ulcerous sore inside the cheek, lips or the gum. Sometimes they are initiated by inadvertently biting the inside of the mouth or by irritation from a denture. Quite often they are indicative of a run-down condition as a result or physical or emotional stress, recovery from illness or as a result of antibiotic treatment.

Treatment

Ensure that your diet is supplying plenty of vitamin C (at least 500 mg daily) and the entire B-complex group. Use the mouthwash recommended above.

Essential Oils: Myrrh, cypress, tea tree.

HAIR PROBLEMS

Falling Hair

Hair loss as a result of stress, certain drugs, illness, malnutrition, dandruff and harsh chemical treatment can eventually be rectified. But it is virtually impossible to restore a healthy head of hair to a man suffering from 'male pattern baldness' which is largely due to the influence of the male hormone testosterone. Baldness in women is relatively rare, and for this reason can be very distressing as society still views female baldness as something of an oddity. If, however, you are a balding man, it may come as some consolation to hear that the surfeit of male hormones surging through your body may arguably make you more masculine than your shock-haired brothers! The female hormone oestrogen, on the other hand, is said to enhance head hair growth which is why many women experience thicker glossier hair during pregnancy when oestrogen levels are high, and why there may be a certain amount of thinning afterwards as a result of hormonal fluctuations.

Healthy hair growth depends on good nutrition, inner

harmony and good scalp circulation. As well as a balanced wholefood diet and a healthy life-style (see Chapter 1) you may need to supplement your diet with brewer's yeast and kelp tablets which are rich in the vital nutrients needed for lustrous hair growth. Obtain your daily quota of protein from eggs, fish, nuts and seeds. Dress salads with a cold-pressed vegetable oil such as olive or sesame and eat plenty of avocados.

Herb Teas: Horsetail, nettle, dandelion.

Having taken care of your diet and life-style, massage your scalp for five to ten minutes every day (described in Chapter 4). Even better results will be achieved if you first comb or brush in one of the hair tonics described in Chapter 5. Yoga, especially the inverted postures (if you can manage them), will encourage a good supply of blood to the hair roots. Otherwise invest in a slant board and lie on it for ten minutes a day with your head downwards to encourage nourishment from the blood to reach your scalp. Shampoo your hair once or twice a week with a mild shampoo containing natural ingredients such as seaweed or nettle extract. Add 4–6 drops of one of the recommended essential oils below to your rinsing water. As a pre-wash conditioner, add six drops of any of the recommended essences to a tablespoonful of coconut, jojoba or almond oil and massage into wet hair and scalp. Wrap your head in a warm towel (replace this every fifteen minutes) and allow the heat of the towel to aid absorption of the oils for about an hour before shampooing. You should only need to carry out this treatment once a week.

Essential Oils: Rosemary, lavender, patchouli.

Dandruff

There are basically two types of dandruff, although derma-tologists may recognise several categories. Simple dandruff (pityriasis) is just dry flaking of the superficial skin cells of the scalp often caused by too little brushing, poor scalp circulation, or use of harsh hair cosmetics and insufficient rinsing out after shampooing. The second kind is fortunately quite rare (seborrheic dermatitis) and appears as thick greasy patches which can easily become infected resulting in scabbing and inflammation. This kind of dandruff is almost certainly the result of a faulty diet or food allergy. Dairy products and of course all 'junk foods' are the main offenders, but it could be an allergy to a seemingly innocent food such as wheat. If you know your diet is well-balanced and you are otherwise healthy and relatively stress-free, it is advisable to have a food allergy test and probably constitutional treatment from a well-qualified homoeopath. However, the treatment outlined here will help both types of dandruff.

Treatment

Similar to the treatment outlined for falling hair, but with a few additions. Medicated shampoos should be avoided like the plague; they tend to clear up the condition for a day or two, but the dandruff returns with a vengeance. If they contain sulphur solutions, rescorcinol, coal tar derivatives and salicylic acid, you may even suffer an allergic reaction causing severe scalp irritation and damaged hair as well. Choose a mild shampoo containing extracts of white nettle or nasturtium. The most beneficial essential oils are camomile, juniper or lavender, to be used in the same way as described for falling hair. For your pre-wash conditioner, add the contents of two vitamin E capsules. It may also be worthwhile taking 4×500 mg of evening primrose oil every day; it has been shown to help many skin disorders, including eczema and dermatitis which are similar to dandruff in many ways.

Other Therapies: Medical herbalism, naturopathy, food allergy testing, homoeopathy.

Essential Oils: Camomile, juniper, lavender, rosemary, tea tree, cedarwood.

HAYFEVER

This is seasonal allergy to airborne pollens or mould spores. Symptoms manifest as excessive sneezing; an itchy, blocked or runny nose; irritated, red watery eyes and sensitivity to light. Some people suffer asthma-like symptoms, causing them to cough or wheeze.

In an allergic person, the body's defence system reacts to pollen as if it were poison, so it produces antibodies which interact with pollen leading to the release of histamine and other chemicals. These cause the classic symptoms of hayfever.

Cause

Although heredity plays a part, hayfever, and allergies in general, are often associated with stress, faulty nutrition, poor posture and shallow breathing.

Treatment

First improve your diet and take steps to reduce some of the stress in your life by relaxation or meditation techniques (Chapter 1). You may find that cutting down on dairy products is helpful; these tend to exacerbate catarrhal conditions. Start your healing regime with a twenty-four hour fast on bottled water and fruit juices (diluted 50/50 with water) followed by a day or two on just grapes or a mixture of fresh fruits (but do seek medical advice first). This will help to eliminate the accumulation of mucus. Increase your vitamin C and B-complex intake. Vitamin C (with added bioflavonoids) is a natural anti-histamine, but must be taken in high doses to work - 4-6 500 mg doses a day. Vitamin B-complex, particularly the B vitamin pantothenic acid, has been shown to reduce stress levels in the body. Lack of B vitamins will intensify allergic reactions. Another helpful supplement is pollen granules. Take half a teaspoonful a day beginning two months before the hayfever season begins.

Yoga, and the special yoga breathing exercises called pranayama, will help to correct poor posture and shallow breathing.

Try garlic capsules; the dosage is 2-4 capsules a day. Aromatic baths and massage with appropriate essential oils will help to reduce your overall stress load. Gradually reduce supplements as improvement takes place.

Herb Teas: Eyebright (this can be used to bathe irritated eyes too), elderflower, goldenseal, elecampane.

Other Therapies: Yoga, autogenics, acupuncture, shiatsu, reflexology, naturopathy, chiropractic or osteopathy (to correct structural faults which may be hindering correct breathing), medical herbalism, Bach Flower Remedies.

Essential Oils: Camomile, eucalyptus, lemon, orange, lavender, garlic (capsules), pine, cypress.

HEADACHE

There are many possible causes of headache far too numerous to mention here, but some of the commonest triggers include nervous tension, high blood pressure, food allergy, muscle spasm at the base of the skull, structural misalignment, constipation, inhalation of toxic fumes and air pollution.

Treatment

First look to your diet and life-style and make the necessary adjustments as outlined in Chapter 1. Dietary and chemical causes will respond readily to corrective measures, but sometimes a food allergy test may be necessary, especially if your headaches could be described more accurately as migraine (see page 159).

Structural faults should be investigated by a chiropractor or an osteopath. However, massage is one of the finest treatments for stress-related headache. If you can find a willing friend or an aromatherapist, so much the better, but the scalp massage described in Chapter 4 will help enormously. Ideally, massage should also include the back (to relax the central nervous system), neck, shoulders and face with the appropriate essential oils. However, do not mix them in a concentration above 1 per cent as the aroma may prove too overpowering and may even exacerbate the problem.

A headache can also be helped by the application of an icy cold compress (Chapter 4) containing peppermint essence.

Herb Teas: Camomile, peppermint, marjoram, skullcap, rosemary.

Other Therapies: Yoga, autogenics, Alexander technique, chiropractic, osteopathy, allergy testing.

Essential Oils: Camomile, lavender, marjoram, peppermint, rose otto, rosemary.

HERPES SIMPLEX (Cold sores)

A painful sore occurring on the lips or around the mouth, brought on by internal toxicity as a result of poor nutrition and stress. The virus lies dormant in many people and only flares up if the body becomes weakened. Herpes can be exacerbated by the sun which can also be a trigger in susceptible people.

Treatment

Look closely to your diet, life-style and emotions (Chapter 1). You may need to take supplementary vitamins for a while, particularly B-complex and vitamin C. Drink horsetail tea *(Equisetum arvense)* three times a day. It is rich in silicon – an aid to herpes (and all skin problem) sufferers. Apply the following lotion three or four times a day: 50 ml distilled water, 1 tsp tincture of myrrh, 4 drops of tea tree essence (or any of those recommended below). Decant into a dark glass bottle and shake well before use.

Other Therapies: Naturopathy, herbalism, homoeopathy.

Essential Oils: Camomile, eucalyptus, myrrh, lemon, tea tree, melissa.

INDIGESTION

The most common forms of indigestion are heartburn, flatulence and abdominal pain.

Cause

Eating too quickly, overeating, incompatible food combinations such as bread with oranges; eating irregularly, nervous tension or food allergy.

Treatment

Investigate the cause, as persistent indigestion may be indicative of something more serious. Adapt your diet and life-style where necessary. For nervous indigestion use any of the following herb teas: camomile, basil, marjoram, melissa. Other tonic and stimulating herbs are fennel, peppermint, spearmint, rosemary, caraway. Aromatic baths and gentle abdominal massage (using circular strokes in a clockwise direction) will be beneficial.

Essential Oils: Fennel, coriander, peppermint, bergamot, marjoram, rosemary, cardamom.

INFLUENZA

The medical textbook definition of 'flu is that the condition is a viral infection that affects the upper respiratory tract. It manifests as symptoms of chills, fever, headaches, general aches and pains and nasal congestion.

The 'flu virus weakens the body's defences against bacteria, and there is a risk of developing a secondary pneumonia. Therefore, it is vital when recovering from 'flu to avoid getting chilled or over-tired through physical exertion of *any* kind - this includes jogging and other energetic sports. The causes are similar to those of colds.

Treatment

As for colds, but with a greater emphasis on eucalyptus or tea tree essence which have marked anti-viral properties. Take four to six garlic capsules daily for a week or more until the acute stage is over, then reduce the dosage to two or three a day during the recovery period which may be as long as a month in some cases.

Essential Oils: Black pepper, eucalyptus, peppermint, rosemary, cypress, lavender, tea tree, cedarwood.

INSECT BITES AND STINGS

Essential oils are almost miraculous in their power to neutralize the poison of insect bites and stings. My favourite stand-by in the summer is a bottle of lavender essence, which can be applied neat. The most important thing to remember is to apply the oil *as soon as possible*. The pain will diminish in a matter of seconds.

Essential Oils: Lavender, lemon, tea tree.

INSOMNIA

We nearly all experience the occasional sleepless night as a result of stress, anxiety, or excitement about the following day. Usually this is short-lived and normal sleep patterns return once the crisis is over. But if insomnia becomes a nightly occurrence, particularly if it leaves you feeling drained the next day, steps must be taken to alleviate the problem safely and naturally.

Do not resort to sleeping pills no matter how desperate you feel. Not only are they physically and psychologically addictive, they do not induce real sleep. Drugged sleep is dreamless. Our dreams are an important emotional safety valve, vital for our mental and emotional equilibrium. People who try to come off regular doses of sleep-inducing drugs too suddenly, experience frightening nightmares or hallucinations as the body desperately tries to catch up on all the dreaming it has been denied. This same phenomenon – 'REM rebound' – occurs when we are continually woken from the dream stage of sleep (signified by rapid eye movement) for several days and then allowed to sleep naturally.

Cause

Insomnia can be linked to many causes; some of the most

common being: a sedentary life-style; lack of fresh air; eating a heavy meal late in the evening; too much tea, coffee or cocoa; nervous tension; or sometimes as a result of nutritional deficiencies. These are often B-complex, vitamin E, zinc and calcium.

Treatment

Changes in diet and life-style (see Chapter 1). If you cannot drop off, read a book, make great plans, but do not just lie there worrying about not being asleep. The more we crave sleep the more likely it is to elude us. No one has yet died of insomnia, but many have become ill through worry.

The following herb teas are renowned for their sleep-inducing properties. They are non-addictive and encourage natural sleep: camomile, californian poppy, hops, meadow-sweet, lime flower, orange flower, passion flower. Valerian tea is probably the most effective, but it does have a foul taste!

Have a warm aromatic bath each evening with one or two of the essences below. After your bath massage the same oils mixed in a vegetable oil into your skin. You might like to sprinkle one or two drops onto your pillow at night or use a hop pillow if you prefer.

By far the most effective treatment for insomnia is a professional aromatherapy massage; many people drop off to sleep before the end of the experience!

Essential Oils: Lavender, camomile, marjoram, clary sage, sandalwood, neroli, rose, ylang-ylang.

THE MENOPAUSE

Sadly, many women dread the onset of the menopause as if it were somehow the beginning of a grey avenue of mental and physical deterioration heightened by the loss of their sexuality and, hence, their worth as women. Such attitudes are fuelled by society's obsession with the cult of youth eternal. Instead of 'growing old gracefully' many women pathetically grab at hormone replacement therapy (HRT), face lifts and stringent diets in an attempt to preserve their youth (men, I hasten to add, are not immune to some of these practices either). Although it would be wrong to rule out HRT completely, very few women really need to take such drastic measures. Reports are appearing in medical literature which suggest that the long-term use of HRT is associated with thrombosis and uterine cancer.

In some African tribes, the cessation of menstrual periods marks the threshold of seniority and rank. Women at this time are given full tribal equality as a mark of gratitude for their many years of child-bearing.

Research suggests that the women who sail through the menopause without any problems at all tend to feel secure in their jobs and relationships, and therefore they feel valued as people. However, it would be wrong to conclude that all menopausal symptoms are caused by our negative attitudes to life. Mind and body are inseparably linked, so hormonal upheavals are bound to cause a certain degree of emotional and physical discomfort. Menopausal symptoms include the 'hot flush' (caused by a rush of hormones into the bloodstream), palpitations, thinning of hair, shrinking of the breasts, vaginal dryness, headaches and many other minor ailments. No wonder women often suffer from irritability, poor concentration and insomnia as well.

Cause

At around 42–50 years of age (sometimes even younger) there is a decreased output of the female sex hormones oestrogen and progesterone. The woman will at first miss one or two periods, eventually the hormone production falls off and periods stop completely.

Treatment

Read Chapter 1 on life-style and diet and supplement this with a good multi vitamin and mineral supplement. Specially formulated 'menopausal' packs are available from chemists and health shops. Pollen has also been found to be effective in reducing menopausal symptoms.

Herb Teas

Black cohosh (a North American herb) and sage. The latter has oestrogen-like properties and can help to reduce the 'hot flushes'.

Aromatherapy treatment should ideally include regular massage to balance the nervous system, but self-treatment with aromatic baths and the application of essences to the skin can be very helpful.

Essences of cypress and sage have the ability to normalise the secretions of female sex hormones and both have a role to play in the treatment of menopausal symptoms. Most authorities recommend camomile, fennel and geranium as well.

Other Therapies: Yoga, acupuncture, medical herbalism, homoeopathy.

Essential Oils: Cypress, clary sage, geranium, camomile, fennel.

MENSTRUAL PROBLEMS

Amenorrhoea (irregular, scanty or cessation of periods)

Surprisingly this may not be a problem at all if we are to believe some of the fascinating evidence being put forward by some of the leading health gurus. In her book *Raw Energy*, Lesley Kenton extols the many virtues of an almost totally raw food diet. It appears that active, *healthy*, lean women on largely vegetarian raw food diets experience fewer, lighter and shorter periods free of pre-menstrual disturbances and pain. Furthermore, it does not appear to affect fertility even though menstruation sometimes ceases altogether on this regime, particularly if the diet is high in bioflavonoids (found naturally in the pith of citrus fruits) and carotene (especially from raw carrots). Feminists, some of whom regard menstruation as one of the many obstacles to women's freedom, may regard this as a revelation! However, I feel it is important to point out that cessation of periods is also symptomatic of chronic illness, particularly of the slimmer's disease *anorexia nervosa*, which results in severe vitamin and mineral deficiencies.

Menstrual upsets can occur as a result of emotional stress of one kind or another. This can include happy experiences such as a foreign holiday or a love affair, as well as trauma. Coming off the pill has been shown to disrupt the menstrual cycle for many months in some women.

Women's periods are measured in approximately 28-day cycles, corresponding to the phases of the moon. However, 'normal' cycles can be shorter or longer than this. (Incidentally, men have cycles too, measured not only by ovulation and blood flow, but by weight loss and change in albumen content of the urine). This moon-related knowledge was used to good effect in the early 1960s by a doctor of physics who had been reading ancient myths and literature on sexual cycles. He decided to experiment with moonlight on women whose menstrual cycles were irregular. By sleeping with the curtains open at night to allow the full rays of the moon to beam in through the window, he found that most of the women ovulated and began to have regular cycles for the first time. Similar experiments using artificial light have been carried out more recently and seem to support this idea. If you decide to try out moonlight for yourself during the summer months, you may discover its only drawback: you could be rudely awakened at some unearthly hour by the bright and cheery masculine rays of the morning sun!

If irregular periods are affecting your fertility, or if they have ceased altogether and you feel emotionally and physically under par, it is advisable to have a medical check-up and to look closely at your diet, life-style and emotions (Chapter 1). Aromatherapy, in conjunction with herbs and a mind/body therapy such as yoga will help to establish a natural rhythm.

Essential Oils: Camomile, clary sage, fennel, melissa, rose.

Dysmenorrhoea (painful periods)

In some women, the cramping pains experienced as the uterus contracts during menstruation can be incapacitating.

Treatment

First look to your diet and life-style (Chapter 1) and supplement your diet with calcium and magnesium tablets (dolomite), or at least for the week prior to your period. These two minerals are known to promote uterine relaxation. In addition to this, drink any of the herb teas listed below. Aromatherapy treatment includes regular massage, particularly to the lower back, aromatic baths, and as a first-aid measure to relieve the cramps, hot compresses over the abdomen. Alternatively, *very gently* apply a massage oil containing camomile or another essence (see below) in a 3 per cent concentration to your abdomen. Then with your fingertips only, stroke downwards over your abdomen with a featherlike touch to soothe and relax the uterus. Heavier pressure is not advisable as it can cause further pain.

Herb Teas: Cramp bark (decoction), caraway, camomile, marigold, chaste tree.

Other Therapies: Yoga, acupuncture, shiatsu, reflexology, medical herbalism.

Essential Oils: Camomile, clary sage, cypress, juniper, marjoram, lemon, rosemary.

Menorrhagia (heavy periods)

Although this condition can be helped with herbs, aromatherapy and diet, you must consult a gynaecologist if the problem persists after several months of natural therapy as it may indicate a more serious problem.

Treatment

British gynaecologist C. Alan B. Clemetson has discovered the relationship between citrus bioflavonoids (found naturally in the pith of citrus fruits) and the reduction of excessive menstrual flow. He recommends high doses of vitamin C with added bioflavonoids (around 4×500 mg daily). Otherwise eat at least three large oranges every day. Bioflavonoids appear to have the ability to compensate for the fall of oestrogen levels occurring three days after ovulation and again just before menstruation. It is partly because of this ability that they help to reduce menstrual flow.

Herbs with a special affinity for the uterus and associated tissues should be drunk three times a day in the week leading up to a period and during the flow itself.

Herb Teas: Cranesbill, periwinkle (lesser), cypress (decoction of the crushed cones).

Aromatherapy treatment includes use of essential oils in your bath and regular aromatherapy massage, particularly to the lower back.

Other Therapies: Medical herbalism, acupuncture, homoeopathy.

Essential Oils: Cypress, geranium, rose.

Pre-Menstrual Syndrome (PMS)

This condition was previously called PMT (pre-menstrual tension); however, 'syndrome' is a more apt term because tension is but one of many other symptoms, both emotional and physical. PMS can begin at any time from two days to two weeks before menstruation. Physical symptoms can include fluid retention, weight gain, bloating, breast tenderness, headaches, nausea, disturbed sleep and skin eruptions. As well as tension, there may be other psychological symptoms such as lethargy, depression, low self-esteem, food cravings, irrational weeping, and irritability. Luckily, very few women suffer all these symptoms, but all women experience some degree of pre-menstrual change.

Before we look at the causes and the treatment of PMS, it is interesting to note that women living in primitive communities very rarely experience PMS, not because they may be healthier, but because they rarely have the opportunity to be pre-menstrual in the first place. During their fertile years they are either pregnant or breastfeeding which can delay menstruation for up to three years. Some degree of pre-menstrual disturbance may be quite a reasonable reaction on behalf of the body to an enforced state of non-pregnancy. Of course it would be ludicrous to suggest that women should give in to biology, heaven forbid, but it is reasonable to accept that menstruation is bound to cause a few *minor* symptoms. No woman, however, should endure severe PMS; short of suppressing menstruation altogether (see 'Amenorrhoea') there is much a woman can do to lessen the symptoms safely and naturally without the need for drugs or hormone treatment.

Cause

There probably is no single cause; a number of feasible explanations have been put forward, ranging from vitamin B6 deficiency to over-production of the hormone prolactin; and from essential fatty acid deficiency to excessively high oestrogen levels in the blood. It appears that fluid retention (whatever the cause of this may be) is responsible for the majority, if not all of the symptoms.

Treatment

First look to your diet and life-style and take steps to reduce the adverse effects of stress by practising a relaxation or meditation technique (see Chapter 1). Evening primrose oil could be an important supplement to your diet. Trials at St Thomas's hospital in London have revealed the oil to be helpful in reducing PMS symptoms. The oil contains gamma linoleic acid (GLA). Too little GLA results in our producing too low a level of cell substances called prostaglandins E1 (PGE1). A deficiency of PGE1 makes a woman's body hypersensitive to tiny changes in hormonal levels. To work efficiently, evening primrose oil is best taken with vitamin B6, B3, zinc, magnesium and vitamin C. There are now 'premenstrual packs' of evening primrose oil, with the above nutrients already added.

The following herb teas are recommended and can be mixed together in equal quantities if you like. The first three are mildly diuretic, but are perfectly safe because they are high in potassium to compensate for any possible loss of the mineral in the urine (one of the drawbacks of standard diuretic drugs). Chaste tree *(Vitex agnus castus)* is capable of normalizing the activity of female sex hormones. It is widely used by medical herbalists to help women with painful periods as well as for pre-menstrual stress.

Herbal Teas: Dandelion, camomile, parsley, chaste tree.

Aromatherapy treatment includes regular massage and aromatic baths with any of the essences listed below. They are all diuretics with relaxant properties, but geranium is particularly helpful to those suffering from a bloated abdomen (or general bloatedness due to fluid retention) and tender breasts.

Other Therapies: Yoga, medical herbalism, Bach Flower Remedies.

Essential Oils: Rose, camomile, cedarwood, cypress, frankincense, geranium, juniper, lavender, sandalwood, patchouli, neroli, ylang-ylang.

MENTAL FATIGUE

This condition does not only afflict the young adults of the family studying for their exams, it is by no means uncommon among harassed mothers and office workers as well.

Treatment

Aromatic baths and inhalations. Put a few drops of any of the recommended essences onto a handkerchief and inhale as required. Rose petal tea is very helpful - a remedy going back to the Romans. Deep breathing exercises should be done as often as possible before an open window or in the fresh air. Best of all is a face, neck and scalp massage - a truly revitalising experience!

Other Therapies: Deep relaxation, meditation, yoga (particularly the inverted postures), Bach Flower Remedies.

Essential Oils: Rosemary, basil, peppermint, coriander.

MIGRAINE

Migraine is very distressing and debilitating headache accompanied by altered vision, nausea and sometimes vomiting.

Cause

There are many possible causes, which may include stress, structural misalignment, muscle spasm at the base of the skull, hormonal disturbance (menopause, the pill) and food allergy. The commonest food triggers are cheese, chocolate, coffee, strong tea, red wine, yeast products, vitamin B supplements, vinegar, animal fat, red meat and sugar. You may not be sensitive to all these substances, but sometimes you may react to an accumulation of one type, or a combination of two or more foods that only cause an attack when the body reaches 'saturation point'. The personality of the sufferer may also be a direct link; they tend to be anxious, hard-working, restless perfectionists.

Treatment

This will require in-depth attention to the cause with the help of a qualified natural therapist such as a medical herbalist, osteopath/naturopath or possibly a homoeopath. Self-treatment is not always successful, especially if the root of the problem is structural misalignment; for this you will certainly need an osteopath or chiropractor. Aromatherapy massage (or massage without essential oils if you are taking homoeopathic medicine) should be used in conjunction with other natural therapies to relieve nervous tension and muscle spasm.

Herb Teas to Help Migraine: If food allergy or poor digestion is at the root of your problem, then choose from the following herbs: camomile, meadowsweet, black horehound, peppermint. If stress is a trigger then choose from the following: skullcap, valerian, vervian, hops. General migraine remedies include feverfew, passion flower, wood betony.

Other Therapies: Food allergy test, osteopathy, chiropractic, naturopathy, acupuncture, shiatsu, reflexology, yoga, meditation, medical herbalism, homoeopathy.

Essential Oils: Camomile, eucalyptus, lavender, marjoram, melissa, peppermint, rosemary.

MUSCULAR ACHES AND PAINS

Massage with the appropriate essential oils will help to alleviate muscle pain caused by over-exertion, poor posture, emotional trauma or rheumatic type aches (see 'Arthritis and Rheumatism'). It is vital, however, to avoid massage if there is any inflammation, swelling or injury, as you may cause even more pain and further damage to body tissue. In such cases, apply a cold compress as first-aid (Chapter 4) followed by a warm compress or massage once swelling and inflammation have disappeared.

Regular massage will improve muscular tone by encouraging a good flow of blood and therefore nutrients to the muscles, thus facilitating optimum function with minimum strain. But do not take this as an excuse to 'go for the burn' as many aerobics enthusiasts have advocated in recent years. This can cause untold damage, leading to . rock-hard muscles and sometimes torn ligaments and tendons as well.

As a preventative therapy, yoga or Alexander technique will correct your posture, relieve emotional as well as physical tension, and encourage efficient use of the body. The techniques are best learned by attending classes, but find a well-qualified and experienced teacher of either practices for them to be of utmost value.

Essential Oils: Bergamot, camomile, camphor, coriander, eucalyptus, lemon, lavender, geranium, marjoram, rosemary, cedarwood.

NIGHTMARES

We all experience bad dreams occasionally, normally after a period of stress or during illness. They should be regarded as an emotional safety valve and not a problem unless they become a habitual pattern (read the section on 'Sleep' in Chapter 1).

Treatment

The same as for anxiety, depression and insomnia. Added to the advice outlined in these sections, you may find it helpful to spray your bedroom (or use an essential oil burner an hour before you go to bed) with any of the recommended essences below. Camomile, however, is generally regarded as a specific and should dominate all your blends.

Herb Teas: Camomile, lime blossom, lemon balm.

Essential Oils: Camomile, lavender, frankincense, sandalwood, rose, neroli.

RINGWORM

A red itchy rash appearing in circular patches anywhere on the body.

Cause

A fungal infection closely related to the athlete's foot fungus. It is exacerbated by poor hygiene and man-made fibres that inhibit the free flow of perspiration. Children often pick up the infection from pets or farm animals.

Treatment

Clothing must be washed thoroughly as the fungus is capable of surviving through the wash and reinfecting the skin. Expose your body to fresh air and sunlight whenever you can. Take three or four garlic capsules a day or include plenty of garlic in your cooking. Apply a cream or ointment (Chapter 5) containing an appropriate essence (see below). You may find it easier to make and use the following lotion: 50 ml distilled water, 1 teaspoon tincture of myrrh, 2 drops tagetes, and 2 drops of geranium, or lavender.

Essential Oils: Tagetes, eucalyptus, geranium, lemon, myrrh, tea tree, lavender, patchouli.

SINUSITIS

This is an infection of the sinus cavities resulting in nasal congestion, pain around the eyes, headaches and sometimes bad breath as well. If not treated properly, the condition can develop into a chronic complaint causing almost constant discomfort.

Cause

Stress, food allergy and air pollution are contributing factors, but the most common cause is a diet too high in mucus-forming foods.

Treatment

Look to your diet and life-style (see Chapter 1) but during the healing period, which can be at least three months, you must drastically reduce all mucus-forming foods. These include dairy products, potatoes, gluten-rich grains such as wheat, rye, barley and oats, sugar and alcohol, and foods laden with additives. Replace these with a largely raw-food diet consisting of fruits, vegetables, bean and seed sprouts, sunflower seeds and juices. Augment this cleaning diet with moderate amounts of high-protein foods such as fish, particularly oily fish, free-range poultry and no more than three eggs a week. It will be helpful to supplement your diet with a good multi-vitamin and mineral supplement and extra vitamin C (4×500 mg a day). Include plenty of raw garlic in your diet or take 2-4 garlic capsules a day.

Herb Teas: Elderflower, eyebright, eucalyptus leaves, peppermint.

Whilst suffering, steam inhalations with any of the essences listed below should be carried out two or three times a day. You can also add any of the essences to your bath. Make up a concentrated massage oil containing four drops of essential oil to each teaspoonful of vegetable oil and rub a very small amount around your nostrils and into your chest at night but not if you have sensitive skin. Alternatively, make up the basic ointment recipe (Chapter 5) and add 15-20 drops of essential oil.

Other Therapies: Naturopathy, medical herbalism, yoga, allergy testing.

Essential Oils: Garlic (internally), eucalyptus, lavender, pine, lemon, peppermint.

SORE THROAT

A sore throat is often the first symptom of a cold or 'flu virus or some other viral infection.

Treatment

Whatever the cause, treatment should include a gargle three times a day with the following mixture: 100 ml distilled water, 5 drops lemon, 5 drops eucalyptus, 5 drops rosemary or clary sage. Shake well before use and use two or three teaspoonfuls of the mixture diluted in a teacupful of warm water.

Essential Oils: Lemon, bergamot, rosemary, eucalyptus, clary sage.

SPRAINS

As soon as possible after the accident apply a cold compress using one of the essences recommended below and renew every hour until the swelling and pain have subsided. Afterwards, apply an ointment (see Chapter 5) containing essential oils to aid hearing.

Essential Oils: Eucalyptus, lavender, camphor, rosemary, tea tree.

TEETHING

If a baby is experiencing problems cutting his or her teeth, you will certainly know about it. He or she will be very irritable and perhaps wakeful during the night, and may cry to be picked up, only to cry to be put down again. One or both cheeks may be flushed and he or she may chew on a fist and drool a lot.

Treatment

Herbalist Jean Palaiseul, author of *Grandmother's Secrets*, swears by marshmallow. He suggests that the baby bites (sucks?) on a piece of the root.

An aromatherapist may suggest rubbing a ½ per cent dilution of camomile essence in almond oil onto the flushed cheek.

Other Therapy: Homoeopathy.

Essential Oil: Camomile.

THREAD VEINS

These are broken capillaries (tiny blood vessels) found just under the surface of the skin. The fine veins become easily dilated, resulting in congestion under the skin which shows up as spidery red streaks particularly on the cheeks and nose where the skin is especially thin.

Cause

Heredity plays a part; but the condition can be caused or made worse by exposure to the elements, strong tea, coffee, tobacco and over-spiced food.

Treatment

Always wear a good protective moisturising cream and avoid facial steams, hot baths and saunas. The best way to strengthen the walls of veins and capillaries is to take 2×500 mg of vitamin C with bioflavonoids daily. Bioflavonoids increase the effectiveness of vitamin C. They are found naturally in citrus fruits and buckwheat. Buckwheat contains the riboflavonoid rutin which is available in tablet form.

Make a facial oil (see Chapter 4) with a proportion of wheatgerm oil and the appropriate essence(s).

Essential Oils: Camomile, cypress, juniper, lemon, rose.

THRUSH (Vaginal)

Thrush is an infection of the mucous membranes of the vagina by the fungus *Candida albicans*, which can also affect the mouth, throat or intestines. Thrush is characterized by a patchy white membranous material giving the affected area a speckled appearance – hence its name 'thrush'. In vaginal thrush, a thick white discharge is present accompanied by intense itching.

Cause

Candida albicans organisms are normal inhabitants of the body and are harmless when the mucous membranes lining the area are healthy. Under certain conditions, however, infection can arise in the areas mentioned above. If the colonies of helpful bacteria are destroyed by antibiotics, for example, the thrush organisms multiply and produce the irritating symptoms. Environmental factors favouring the growth of the fungus include warmth, moisture, sugar and yeast in the diet, and alkaline vaginal secretions as a result of the pill. Thrush can occur due to reinfection during intercourse. Men can carry the infection as a result of intercourse with a woman suffering from thrush, or following antibiotic treatment; but they are often free of symptoms.

Treatment

This is largely dietary. Drastically reduce your sugar, yeast and alcohol consumption and follow a well-balanced wholefood diet as described in Chapter 1. Take 3–4 garlic capsules daily (garlic has antifungal properties) and drink copious amounts of bottled spring water and any of the herb teas recommended below. It is helpful to take lactobacillus acidophilus tablets (but they are expensive) or to eat 300 ml of plain live yoghurt a day until the attack is over. You may also need to supplement your diet with a good multi-vitamin and mineral formula, or with a yeast-free B-complex supplement.

Avoid wearing nylon tights or knickers and very tight jeans. These do not allow the air to circulate, thus trapping perspiration and creating the ideal environment for *Candida* to flourish.

Aromatic baths containing any of the essences below should be taken daily during an attack.

Herb Teas: Camomile, nettle, blackberry (leaves).

Other Therapies: Medical herbalism, naturopathy, homoeopathy.

Essential Oils: Lavender, garlic (taken in capsule form), geranium, lemon, cedarwood, tea tree.

TONSILLITIS

The tonsils are two small lumps of lymphatic tissue, one on each side of the throat at the base of the tongue. Their role, in common with other lymphatic glands, is to defend the body from infection. Inflammation and enlargement of the tonsils – tonsillitis – is the body's attempt to throw off toxins.

Treatment

Natural treatment aims to support the body in its attempt to restore balance. Surgery to remove the tonsils is seldom a wise decision. Future minor toxicity crises will cause more discomfort by inflammation of the throat and 'flu-like symptoms.

A 24-hour fast or semi-fast on grapes and grape juice is the best approach, but do seek medical advice. Drink plenty of spring water and take a cup of the herbal brew recommended below, three times a day. Gradually move on to a largely raw diet (but read the precautions outlined in the dietary section in Chapter 1). During the fast it is important to rest to allow the body's healing processes to work unimpaired.

Herbal Tea: Mix equal quantities of the following herbs and make a herb tea according to the instructions on page 109. Red sage, horehound, marigold.

Add any of the recommended essences to your bath. Rub a 3 per cent concentration of geranium into the throat area (but not if you have sensitive skin). Using a special hand spray (available from pharmacists), regularly spray your throat with lemon juice diluted 50/50 with water or add 5 drops of the essence to 150ml water.

Other Therapies: Homoeopathy, medical herbalism, naturopathy.

Essential Oils: Geranium, lemon, bergamot.

TOOTHACHE

Apply one or two drops of essential oil directly into the tooth cavity; repeat as often as necessary until you can see your dentist. Prevent tooth decay in the first place by good nutrition and scrupulous dental hygiene (see also 'Gums').

Essential Oils: Camomile, clove (dilute 50:50 with vegetable oil), peppermint.

VARICOSE VEINS

These are swollen, knotted veins, usually in the legs, but they can occur elsewhere in the body.

Cause

Obesity, lack of exercise, constipation, prolonged standing, insufficient fluid intake and a toxic diet.

Treatment

A wholefood diet and adequate exercise. The best exercises are walking and swimming. Yoga is extremely beneficial too, especially the inverted postures. You must rest with your feet higher than your head for about 10 minutes every day. You may find that sleeping with your bed slightly elevated on blocks at the foot-end can be even more helpful.

The following supplements will help: 4×500 mg vitamin C, a good vitamin E supplement and a good bioflavonoid supplement called rutin. Rutin is found naturally in buckwheat tea and in the pith of citrus fruits. Together with vitamin C, rutin will help to relieve pain and swelling and will strengthen the capillary walls.

Cypress essence will help to diminish the varicosity if massaged *gently* over the veins every day. Use upward strokes to encourage the circulation back to the heart. Mix the essence into the cream or ointment recipe in Chapter 5, or make a massage oil.

Other Therapies: Herbalism, naturopathy.

Essential Oils: Cypress, lemon.

VERRUCAE (plantar warts)

These are ingrowing warts found on the ball of the foot caused by a viral infection. The treatment is the same as for ordinary warts (see below).

WARTS

Small, hard growths on the skin most commonly found on the hands, but they can occur on other parts of the body. Those occurring on the ball of the foot are called verrucae (ingrowing warts) and are treated in the same way.

Cause

A viral infection. Stress, as well as poor nutrition, lowers our resistance to all types of infection.

Treatment

Ensure that your diet is rich in all nutrients (Chapter 1) particularly vitamin B-complex, C and E. You may need to supplement your diet with these during the healing period. To reduce stress, practise a conscious form of relaxation such as meditation, deep relaxation or perhaps yoga. Garlic is a lymphatic cleanser and tonic capable of boosting the immune system and should be taken internally as garlic capsules. Take up to four a day for a month or two.

Externally, apply neat lemon essence. Put one or two drops on the gauze portion of a plaster and apply over the wart. Change the dressing daily, but always remove at night to allow the skin to breathe. It may take a week or about a month for the wart to shrivel and fall away. If the skin has become dry and flaky after the lemon essence treatment, apply the contents of a vitamin E capsule or some wheatgerm oil to the area. Vitamin E, found naturally in wheatgerm oil, has been found to inhibit the formation of warts, so this is a preventative remedy as well as a cosmetic treatment.

Essential Oils: Garlic, lemon, tea tree.

WOUNDS, CUTS AND GRAZES

Essential oils have powerful antiseptic and healing properties. They are harmless to tissue and do not sting as much as harsh chemical antiseptics.

Serious wounds where there is profuse bleeding should always be treated by a doctor, so get help *immediately*. Meanwhile, apply a bandage that has been sprinkled with lemon oil (it arrests bleeding) and secure tightly.

General cuts and grazes should first be cleaned with lavender oil (6 drops in 300 ml of water). Get as much dirt, grit and any foreign bodies out of the wound as you can. Then apply a piece of lint that has been sprinkled with a mixture of lavender and lemon (or any other essence recommended below) and bandage into place. Smaller wounds can be treated with a plaster. Put the essence onto the gauze portion.

Essential Oils: Lavender, eucalyptus, camomile, geranium, patchouli, juniper, rosemary, frankincense, bergamot, camphor, lemon, tea tree.

Appendix

Useful Addresses

Essential Oil Suppliers
Butterbur and Sage
101 Highgrove Street
Reading RG1 5EJ

Neal's Yard USA
284 Connecticut Street
San Francisco
California 94107

Aromatherapy Courses and Oils
Purple Flame Aromatics
61 Clinton Lane
Kenilworth
Warwickshire CV8 1AS

International Federation of
    Aromatherapists
Stamford House
2–4 Chiswick High Road
London W4 1TH

Institute of Traditional Herbal
    Medicine and Aromatherapy
'The Roses', Studridge Lane
Speen, Princes Risborough
Buckinghamshire HP27 0SF

Dr Edward Bach Healing Society
644 Merrick Road
Lynbrook
New York 11563

Massage Courses
Clare Maxwell-Hudson
87 Dartmouth Road
London NW2 4BR

Kittywake Oils
Cae Kitty, Taliaris
Llandeilo
Dyfed SA19 7DP

Aroma Vera Inc.
PO Box 3609
Culver City
California 90231

Shirley Price Aromatics
Wesley House
Stockwell Head
Hinckley
Leicestershire LE10 1RD

American Society of Phytotherapy
    and Aromatherapy
PO Box 3679
South Pasadena
California 91031

Berida Manor
PO Box 350
Bowral
New South Wales 2576
Australia

Herbs and Cosmetic Materials
Baldwins
171–3 Walworth Road
London SE17

Recommended Reading

AROMATHERAPY
Aromatherapy For Everyone, Robert Tisserand, Arkana 1990
Fragrant Pharmacy, V. A. Worwood, Bantam Press 1990

MASSAGE
The Book of Massage, foreword by Clare Maxwell-Hudson,
   Ebury Press 1984

BABY MASSAGE
Loving Hands, Frederick Leboyer, Collins 1977

HERBAL
The New Holistic Herbal, David Hoffmann, Element Books
   1991

YOGA
Yoga, Cheryl Isaacson, Thorsons 1990

RELAXATION
The Book Of Stress Survival, Alix Kirsta, Gaia Books 1986

HEALTH, BEAUTY AND NUTRITION
The Joy Of Beauty, Leslie Kenton, Century Publishing 1983

Index